FINDING THE *Best* DANCE INSTRUCTION: *Look Before you Leap*

by

BARBARA EARLY

Foreword by

MARGE CHAMPION

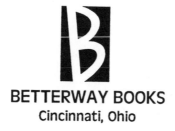

BETTERWAY BOOKS
Cincinnati, Ohio

Cover design by Chris Broquet, CAB Design
Cover photo by Tom Fezzey
Text photos by Tom Fezzey
Typography by Park Lane Associates

97 96 95 94 93   5 4 3 2 1

Library of Congress Cataloging-in-Publication Data

Early, Barbara.
    Finding the best dance instruction : look before you leap /
Barbara Early.
        p. cm.
    Includes index.
    ISBN 1-55870-259-8 : $8.95
    1. Dancing--Study and teaching. I. Title.
GV1589.E27 1992
792.8'07--dc20   92-16484
                                                                   CIP

For those who live to teach dance,
my children who keep me dancing,
and
Tom, whose love lets me dance happily through life!

Acknowledgments

I wish to thank the following people for their invaluable contributions. Their expertise, support, and generosity made this book a reality.

Carol Aldridge, Wagner Community Center
V.F. Beliajus
Jerry Brondfield, Author
Michelle Clyne, Philip J. Rock Center & School
Country Dance and Song Society
Rosemary Doolas, Chicago Dance Medium
Debi Elfenbien, Dance Horizons
Mignon Furman, Royal Academy of Dancing
Debra Goldman, MA, ADTR
David Hoctor, Professional Dance Teachers Association
Luke Kahlich, National Dance Association
Jane Caryl Miller, The Cecchetti Council
Pat Morgan
K.C. Patrick
Vickie Sheer, Dance Educators of America
Paul Wing, Bernie Swartz, and John Guzzarde
Paul Zimmerman, Dance Masters of America

and the wonderful research librarians at the Lisle, Illinois Public Library.

My gratitude goes to "Kay Clay International" and "All That Jazz" for supplying shoes; L'uomo Tuxedo for the tuxedo; and to Utica Dance Center, The School of the Von Heidecke Ballet, and The Bryant Ballet for letting me invade their space.

Thanks to the following family, friends, and dancers who gave of their time and talents to be photographed:

My Children—Jamie Early, Amanda and Matthew Fezzey

and

Michael J. Armstrong
Amanda Baez
Brendan Baker
Monica Lee Blackett
Homer Bryant
Rose Elvey
Mario Ford
Signe Green
Ashera Grossett
Jennifer Guzzarde
Patrick Harvey
Kathy Hasty
Terrence Hasty
Neal Hopkins
Janet N. Houk
Lamar Jefferson
Mary Lou Kelly
Blossom S. Kenis
Brett Kielman
Rachel Krawczyk

Mary Mackin
Laura Mawhinney
Randi Mayor
Lisa Nichols
Michelle Nikonchuk
Mae E. Phipps
Britt Posmer
Shaw Powell
Barbara Rabie
Jeffrey Rausa
Keir Rogers
Cynthia Savage
Remy Schultz
Antonio Strong
Derrick Strong
Erick Strong
Jasmine Thorne
Ralph Valatka
Jon Westgaard

Akasha Dance Company: Terry Bellamy, April M. Brown, David Gomez, Oliver Ramsey, and Laura Wade

and my dance soul mate, Trudi Green-Gavin.

Special thanks to Chris Broquet, designer and friend, for the perfect cover, and to my incredibly talented husband, Tom Fezzey, Photographer.

Foreword

Barbara Early has compiled and written the book I always thought I'd write. No, I felt was absolutely necessary to write!

Growing up in my father's dancing school in Los Angeles in the '20s and '30s, I was given the best of training by the best of teachers. Not only was Ernest Belcher a superb role model and a teacher of teachers, but he gathered around him an incomparable staff for his University of Dance: Edwardo and Elisa Cansino for Spanish, Arthur Prince and Louis da Pron for Tap, and a number of masters in acrobatics, gymnastics, and ballroom dancing. He had been schooled in England by the most renowned Cecchetti and English style ballet masters. His knowledge of the body was as skilled as his knowledge of ballet, ballroom, and Spanish technique. His school was my second home for almost fifteen years of my life. It would have been bad form for me to go shopping around and visiting other schools. I was very fortunate indeed. I was trained under his extraordinary physical and creative tutelage, and my growing body was never threatened by premature, hasty, ignorant methods. My young legs were strengthened thoroughly before pointe shoes were allowed. My personality was nurtured slowly, so that any possibility of precociousness or a case of the "cutes" was largely avoided. Until I was sixteen and a high school graduate, my only brushes with professional appearances were in carefully monitored concerts at the Redlands Bowl, the Hollywood Bowl, and the Greek Theatre. My three-year working arrangement with Walt Disney (as the live action model for Snow White, the Blue Fairy in *Pinocchio*, and the Hippos and Storks in *Fantasia*) was approved because of my father's association with "Uncle" Walt and the total absence of public display of me as a performer "until I was ready."

Little wonder that, until I was quite mature, I would be unaware of the thoughtless and/or greedy practices of some other schools for young performers. Occasionally I'd hear my father grumbling about the bulging calf muscles or overextended back and hip placement of some of the "new" pupils who came to him from other primary teachers. But it was not until later that I came to realize the full extent of the damage that can be visited on a youngster by improper supervision. By the time I was trying my wings in the New York theater in my twentieth year, I also saw the personality damage that could be done by encouraging the premature sexual and super-energized behavior so prevalent in schools ill-prepared to properly nurture a budding talent. Broadway choreographers quickly dismiss any applicants with "recital smiles" no matter how many pirouettes they whip off, and it matters very little if 95% of those enrolled in the thousands of American dancing academies will ever be professional material. What matters is the health and growth of the student and his or her ability to appreciate and enjoy a lifetime experience with the performing arts. If I had chosen a life of raising four children or running a drug store (as my mother did), it would have been immeasurably enriched by my early education under the watchful eye of the Dean of the West Coast Dance Masters. The luck that enabled me to become the partner of Gower Champion, to dance and act and choreograph my way through fifty-five years of show business, was only matched by the luck of having had the right training. I was ready when luck knocked on my door.

And now, I've had the luck of *not* having to spend months of my golden years researching and educating the public in how to choose the RIGHT school and how to avoid the dangerously wrong ones! As I said, Barbara Early has done it brilliantly for me and for you. I am deeply grateful for this much-needed source of knowledge. It may just give you or your children a fair and healthy chance to enhance the quality of whatever life you choose.

Marge Champion
Stockbridge, Massachusetts
1991

Contents

PART IV.
DANCE FOR SPECIAL PEOPLE AND GROUPS

PART V.
WORDS OF WISDOM

Introduction

Do you think that a "ballet barre" is where dancers go to have a beer after class or that "alignment" is something you should only worry about with your car? Do you think ballet students wear their hair up and pink tights as a fashion statement? If so, then you're not alone.

The world of dance is as foreign to most people as outer space. This lack of dance knowledge would not be a problem if people weren't blindly throwing away millions of dollars annually on inadequate, unsafe dance instruction. Thousands of people make their choice of teacher or facility armed with nothing more than their checkbooks. They assume that they are getting competent instruction because studios have local popularity and large enrollments.

The shocking reality is that *anyone* can open up a dance studio or teach classes. They don't need to know anything about anatomy, physiology, professionalism, theater, or even dance for that matter. They only need to convince you that they do. In this day and age when intelligent consumers spend more time researching the quality of their aerobic shoes than the qualifications and credentials of the person who is twisting and bending their children's bodies, is it any wonder that mediocre dance studios grow and prosper? It's shocking!

A child can spend years "studying" with one of these teachers only to find out that she doesn't have a fraction of the training needed to pursue her dreams in dance. In many cases, parents are literally throwing hard-earned dollars out the window and getting glorified day care instead of safe technical instruction. Saddest of all, growing numbers of dance students, children and adults alike, suffer lasting bodily injury under the tutelage of unqualified instructors. All this can be avoided.

You and your child don't have to be a statistic. This guide

cuts through the hype and myths and gives you the basic knowledge required to make an intelligent choice. Whether you are young or old, male or female, able or disabled, headed for Broadway or going for fun, you are entitled to the best dance instruction available. It's out there and you can find it. The world of dance is not that complex. You just have to learn a few of the local customs and speak a little of the language.

I am going to be your interpreter so that you can have a safe, enjoyable, first-rate journey *and* get your money's worth.

No matter where you are in your dance instruction, this guide will be invaluable. If you or your child are currently enrolled in dance classes, it will either validate the instruction you have been receiving or shock you when you discover you've been taken for a ride. If you are contemplating taking classes, it will give you the tools to make a competent selection of a teacher and facility. If you want to make dance your career, it will help guide you through all the phases of dance and give you invaluable advice from real working dance professionals and stars to help you realize your dreams. And if you are a dance teacher or studio owner, this book is the perfect "handout" for your students and will serve as a reference and constant source of inspiration to you and your staff for validating the quality dance training that you are committed to give.

Dance has enlightened my life. I hope that this guide will enlighten yours!

PART I

Finding
the Right Facility

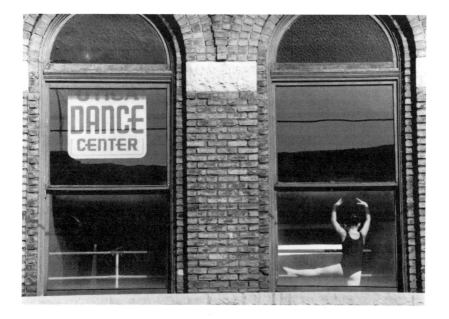

1
What Are Your Options?

The difficulty in life is the choice.
George More

Dance classes are offered in many different settings. Finding out which facility is right for you, or where a certain type of class is being offered, can be confusing to say the least. Let's talk about options.

When you first contemplate instruction for yourself or your child, you automatically think of the neighborhood "dance studio." Most dancers begin their training in just such a place. Under this dance studio umbrella, however, are many different types of facilities offering a wide variety of instruction. In order to make some sense out of all the different studios, I have devised a very general system of classification. There are many, many exceptions in each category and, at the outset, I offer my apology to any studio owner whose nose might get out of joint because of my methods.

I have also made a simplified scale concerning class levels. The difficulty of a class depends entirely on the ability and comprehension of the *majority* of the students. A beginner class at one studio could easily be an intermediate level at another. For clarification purposes, I have broken down the levels into two basic categories — student and professional — with each having three divisions of beginner, intermediate, and advanced. I have also added a "predance" level at the very beginning to cover classes for preschool-age children. I then numbered them

consecutively 0-6; 0 being the very, very raw beginner and pro-
gressing in difficulty until you reach level 6 — the advanced
classes for working professionals. In the real world, you will
find many levels in between (advanced beginner, beginning intermediate, etc.), but for the sake of simplicity and to save my
sanity they are not used here.

TYPES OF DANCE SCHOOLS

Neighborhood Studio

This is the local dance school in a commercial building or
operating out of someone's home. The quality varies greatly in
these studios due to the naiveté of the clientele, and it is here
that a lot of the problems exist. These facilities can run the gamut
from schools that are total wastes of time and money to professional academies with the highest standards. It is absolutely necessary that you screen the teachers carefully because a studio is
only as good as its teachers. These facilities offer a wide variety
of classes and teach ballet, tap, jazz, pointe, modern, ballroom,
and ethnic. Levels range from 0-4, and they teach children and
adults. This is the place where most dancers first fall in love
with dance, and a quality studio can give a student a firm and
lasting foundation.

The more serious schools teach all year long, but many stay
open nine months out of the year and close during the summer.
There is usually an annual or biannual recital or production,
and costume costs are incurred by the participating students or
their parents. The higher quality institutions generally put on
shows every other year to allow for concentrated technique and
training in the "off year." Their productions are usually extensive
and topnotch and sometimes even include singing and acting.

Competition Studios

This is a neighborhood studio where participation in numerous dance competitions is emphasized. You will recognize it
by the trophies and ribbons everywhere. These studios generally spend their "class time" learning routines rather than technique. (So many trophies, so little time!) There could be a lot of
extra costs (i.e., costumes, entry fees, transportation to contests)

and additional rehearsal time. These studios offer the same types of classes as the neighborhood studio, and the levels are 0-3 with classes for children and adults.

Specialty Studios

These schools specialize in a certain type of dance (ballet and pointe, ethnic) and are usually very knowledgeable in their particular area of expertise. The ballet schools can be of a student level or professional caliber and usually have their own performing company or are associated with a major ballet troupe. Caution should be advised when selecting a ballet teacher, however, because there are rotten apples in the barrel, and teachers of this form of dance need special knowledge (see Chapter 8). The levels range from 0-6 and all ages take instruction.

Professional Schools

These are the studios where the "big guns" take and teach class and where the serious student eventually needs to dance. They are usually located in or near major cities, and their curriculum includes ballet, tap, jazz, pointe, and modern. Teachers are almost always professionals, and many are major choreographers. Remember, however, that a dance career doesn't necessarily make a person a good teacher. It can only enhance the abilities of one who is blessed with the gift. Always try to observe the teacher in action, no matter how renowned (see Chapter 4).

Levels 1-6 are taught, and most classes are for students in their teens and up. Some do teach younger children, usually on the weekends.

Academic/Performing Arts Schools

You have probably seen the movie *Fame* and are vaguely familiar with the High School for the Performing Arts in New York. This is the type of facility that falls under this heading. Basically, such schools offer both an academic education and concentrated dance instruction (plus voice and music) all under the same roof. These schools, of which there are only a handful, are *only* for the dedicated dancer who is serious about a performing career. Admission is usually by audition only, and tuition is generally substantial, though scholarships are available. Not for the timid!

Franchise Schools and National Chains

These facilities generally teach recreational "social dancing," and they cater mainly to adults. The levels range from 1-4, and sometimes the lessons are "one on one" with an instructor of the opposite sex. The group lessons can be a great way of socializing but beware of those that require you to sign contracts! Don't sign your life and checkbook away.

TUITION AND HIDDEN COSTS

Speaking of checkbooks, let's talk about tuition rates. Each facility may have different ways of charging for lessons, and the costs vary according to the length of the class. Some studios give discounts if you take more than one class per week or if other members of the same family are also enrolled at the school. It is the norm for studios to require complete payment up-front for an entire month's or semester's worth of classes. That policy assures the teacher that you are making a commitment and also compensates the instructor for his or her time and talents should you withdraw abruptly, leaving a vacancy that cannot be filled.

Don't confuse this good business policy with signing a contract. Once the time period for which you paid for instruction has lapsed, there are no other monetary obligations on your part. If you decide not to show up for a class and you do not take a makeup class (a standard studio practice), you are the loser because you forfeit your tuition. Under a contract situation, however, you could find yourself locked into classes and payments for many months after you have put your signature on a contract and, in many cases, long after you have completed your instruction. Know what you are buying!

Providing a guide to the actual amount of money you should pay per class is difficult if not almost impossible, as it will vary according to areas of the country and other factors. The value of the dollar is a matter of opinion; however, I don't think that any studio should get away with highway robbery. If a professional in New York or Los Angeles can take a class that lasts anywhere from an hour to an hour and a half, from a highly respected teacher of superior caliber, for about $10 (1992 price), then a neighborhood dance studio should not charge nearly that much. Of course, the value of anything can only be determined by the value you place on it. If you believe that you are getting your money's worth and that the training you are receiving is invaluable, then more power to you. You really cannot put a price on good, safe training, and teachers will always charge what the market will bear.

Discounts

Though instruction can be quite costly, there are many discounts available, which you should certainly look into. Most studios will give a price break to seniors, and due to the shortage of male dancers, many will give a healthy discount to men and boys. Rather than putting up with the tedious task of writing weekly receipts, some studios also offer "class cards." A student can purchase a card entitling him to participate in a specified number of classes (usually of his choice), and the card is then stamped or punched each time a class is taken. To make it more appealing, the actual cost for each individual class is usually discounted.

Discounts are sometimes available to people who are in "The Biz." Professional schools sometimes offer a special rate for dance students who are members of theatrical and film unions (i.e., Screen Actors Guild [SAG], American Federation of Television and Radio Artists [AFTRA], and Actors' Equity Association [AEA]). This comes under the heading of professional courtesy.

Dance schools also have an "off season," and just like the travel business will occasionally offer special reduced rates during the summer months.

In an effort to attract gifted students, some studios offer scholarships. I have even seen students and parents with gumption barter for classes. In fact, around the age of twelve when my mother no longer wanted to pay for my instruction, I worked at the studio I attended to pay for the lessons myself. I would answer the phone, clean the mirrors, mop the floors, or whatever was needed, just to be able to dance. I have known many a mom who has sat at the reception desk or sewn on thousands of sequins to give her child a chance at attaining her dream. Most teachers will bend over backward to accommodate a student who has passion or talent or both, so where there is a will there is a way! All you have to do is ask. All of the above are worth investigating and could save you a considerable amount of money in the long run.

Other Fees

There are other potential fees that you should be aware of before you make a decision to sign up for classes. I am referring to the costs of "the recital." Like it or not, the majority of dance schools have a yearly recital or show of some sort, and these productions can be extremely costly to the consumer in terms of both time and money. You need to ask questions and find out before you sign up what you may be getting yourself or your child into. Of course, you don't have to participate in the show, but believe me, not performing in the show is sometimes more difficult than being in it. Let me set the stage for you ...

Your little Susie has been taking dance lessons since September. It is now January and her teacher informs everyone that she will now begin teaching the recital routines in preparation for the June show. The studio will need a $40 deposit for each costume, and Susie's class will be doing two numbers. That's eighty bucks (but who's counting?)! After you regain consciousness, you tell her that Susie might not be able to be in the show. She replies by saying that is fine, but the class will be working exclusively on the recital choreography (so that everyone will be perfect) and Susie is welcome to learn the routine. (Isn't that generous?) Susie will have to stand at the back of the group, of course, so as not to mess up their formations. Now, let's be realistic! Are you really going to have the heart to refuse Susie permission to be in the show? You certainly don't want her to be excluded and feel inferior, and pulling her out of the studio would be throwing months of lessons right down the drain so ... you sign the permission slip and cough up the $80. A few months go by and letters start arriving from the studio concerning additional costs such as makeup, shoe dye, tights, the balance due on those two costumes, studio pictures, show videos, and tickets for the performance (which you have to pay to see). While you are in shock, you add up the number of tickets you will need for family, relatives, and friends, and you take out a second mortgage on your house. (Some studios may only charge a modest admission fee of two to three dollars, but I recently heard a horror story of a local dance school that charges $32.50 a ticket!) On top of all this, there will be added rehearsal times (which the students must attend or risk being thrown out of the cast), and the teacher wants you to volunteer your time to do everything from sewing on fringe to being an usher. It all really is a production. Isn't it?

The Recital Problem

This scenario has become the norm. Of course, there are schools that do things differently, but believe me, studios without some sort of recital are definitely in the minority. You need to find out what the norm is at the studio or facility you are considering *before* you or your child have made an emotional commitment. As long as you know approximately what extra costs will be coming your way, you can be prepared for them. Now you are probably asking yourself if recitals are even necessary. Let me say this for the record: recitals *are not* a necessary part of dance education! There are many other performing outlets that can give a student the stage skills that are needed, and these alternatives won't send you to the poorhouse. The problem with many dance schools today is that the recital has become the "reward" for taking classes. *The satisfaction of knowing how to dance should be a reward in and of itself.* Because of this shift in goals, dance education in the average community studio has become more of a recreational amusement than the study of a serious art form. Many studios offer very little more than recreational babysitting. The focus in these schools is on the "show," which is the biggest advertisement and money maker for the studio, rather than on the teaching of technique. The teachers sometimes spend the entire year (or at least half of it) drilling and drilling cutesy routines. With lessons lasting only half an hour or an hour, there isn't really much time left for actual dance education.

Smart studio owners and concerned dance educators have compromised by having productions every other year, so that they can get in a good year or so of training between shows. This strengthens their students' technique and makes the quality of their shows much more palatable, yet still caters to those students and parents who want recitals. Some have even eliminated recitals altogether and found other performing outlets for their students, such as lecture demonstrations or local theater productions, or by forming their own dance companies. They realize that though it is incredibly important for dance students to have performing experience, the students cannot perform effectively without solid technical training.

If I could change the structure of studios, I would change all shows to biannual productions, and I would only let the intermediate and advanced students participate. This would not only give us better dancers (by giving students more time to master their craft between productions), it would keep parents from incurring added expenses until their children are a little more committed. It would also give beginner students a goal to work toward and would make it a lot less painful for the members of the recital audience. (How many times have you had to suffer through a terminally long, unorganized, boring recital filled with uncoordinated raw beginners?) But I will probably never get my way, so as a consumer, you are going to be faced with the recital dilemma. Good luck!

Competitions

There is another performance outlet that could make an even bigger hole in your pocketbook. It's competitions! Studios have gone crazy for these contests in recent years, and there are big prizes, trophies, and titles at stake. If you think that recitals are expensive, just wait until you get sucked into participating in competitions. Costumes can cost hundreds of dollars, rehearsal times can be all-consuming, and then there are the added expenses of entry fees, transportation costs (usually to a site out of state), hotels, meals, etc. I know of one school so involved in competitions that their precision group is so prestigious, parents pay $1,500 a year (yes, $1,500) for their children to be in it! When it comes right down to it, you have to decide what you want out of a studio and what you are willing to pay for. Just be aware of the vast differences in the goals in dance schools, so that you get the education you really want. Ask up front what the objective of each school is and spend your money accordingly.

The Power of Advertising

This seems like as good a time as any to give you an important warning. *Don't* be impressed by slick studio brochures filled with accolades, adjectives, and promises. When I began doing in-depth research of dance facilities, I received a glut of promotional materials. I was amazed at the stirring contents of the brochures. If I were not familiar with dance and theater, I would have certainly been bowled over by the so-called "credits" of most of the teachers. Knowing, however, which credits really constitute an achievement in the dance world and which, if any, would certify someone to teach dance, I was able to determine quickly that a great many of the dance studio brochures were full of bunk!

Teacher training (or lack thereof) was embellished (to put it mildly), making the majority of teachers sound like ballet masters, prima ballerinas, doctors, or Broadway stars. In actuality, many of these so-called experts were nothing more than advanced beginner or intermediate students themselves. On the other side of the coin, many teachers who had impressive credentials were mediocre instructors at best.

I don't really know how to keep you from being influenced by expensive promotional material, but you *must not* make your choice of facility or teacher on the information in these brochures alone. You have to tread carefully, not take their advertising at face value, and to coin a phrase—Look Before You Leap! The key is to observe the actual teacher and students and take a good long look at the end results. Do you want yourself or your child to dance like their students? If not, or if you want better training, take your business elsewhere.

OTHER ALTERNATIVES

The dance studio setting is not the only place to receive dance training. Many communities offer extensive classes through their Park & Recreation programs and Adult Education. These are no-frills classes, generally held at community centers and public schools. Though they may lack the equipment (barres and mirrors), the classes can still be beneficial if the teacher really knows his or her stuff, and these sessions are very reasonably priced. There is a wide variety of class offerings; however, the levels usually fall within the 0-1 range. As always, check out the teacher's credentials and be extra cautious of the flooring (see Chapters 3 and 4). Community classes are almost always recreational in nature, but they are a good way for children and adults to sample different dance forms inexpensively before taking the studio plunge.

The local YMCA or comparable facility is also a good place to start. Some centers offer the additional benefits of on-site day care or baby-sitting services, and the "perks" that go along with membership (pools, whirlpools, saunas, etc.) make an attractive package for adults. The types of classes that are offered are pretty limited, and the levels are low (0-1), but as long as the teacher is qualified, these simple classes can create a spark in a novice student that can be the beginning of a fiery, lifelong passion for dance.

Community colleges and major universities are a great source for adult dance instruction, and almost all offer some credit and non-credit classes for the recreational dancer or an extensive curriculum for the dancer who wants an academic teaching degree. You will find courses in ballet, jazz, tap, ethnic, ballroom, and comprehensive modern dance. It is within these academic walls that modern dance really flourishes. The teachers are usually people with dance or theater degrees or advanced students who are pursuing their own teaching careers. Though most of the classes are for adults, many universities offer beginning level classes for young children at a minimal cost. The overall levels range from 0-4, and the quality of the instruction is generally top-notch.

With the invention of video, there has arisen yet another interesting option—self-instruction. Nothing can take the place of an actual dance class, but some home videos can be fun and entertaining. They should, however, be used only as a supplement to good class instruction. A beginner needs constant correction and guidance, and there is no way that a dance student can get what she needs from a video. Once a student progresses to a reasonable level of expertise in dance, videos can be a good source of choreographic inspiration, but as teaching tools, they are potentially very dangerous. This is especially true when it comes to ballet and jazz. These two dance forms need continual supervision by an expert to prevent injury. Tap, on the other hand, can be successfully *introduced* by way of video, but there is only a limited amount of knowledge that can be conveyed. If you really want to learn, you will have to turn off the VCR, put your inhibitions aside, and go to a real dance class. I promise you will be glad you did.

OTHER DETERMINING FACTORS

Given all the above information, there may still be other factors that dictate where you take instruction. Most people do not have all the aforementioned facilities to choose from. In rural areas for instance, there may be only one dance studio and instructor. If you are faced with this situation and, if after investigation you find that the facility and teacher in question are only adequate at best, you will have to arm yourself with knowledge to protect yourself from injury and to enhance your dance education. The best way to gain this knowledge is to read. Even the smallest of libraries has a wealth of information on dance terminology, physiology, sport injuries, theater, dance history, music, etc. Absorb this information and apply it to your own particular class and dance experiences.

Workshops

Dance workshops are also invaluable, especially to the suburban student, and their whereabouts, dates, and costs can be found in monthly dance publications. The most extensive periodical of this sort is *Dance Magazine*, which your teacher probably receives. It can also be found in most libraries or can be subscribed to by mail (33 West 60th Street, New York, NY 10023). Workshops advertise regularly in this magazine, so anyone with a mail box can get the needed information. Workshops are held all over the country, usually in major cities, and offer student instruction at many different levels; however, it is usually more beneficial for the attendees to be of at least an intermediate level. The fees for these seminars vary considerably depending on the length, location, number of classes offered, and reputations of the teachers, but most sessions are well worth the time and money. Exposure to students from different areas and with varied backgrounds can rapidly put things into perspective and can help a student set goals, redefine her level of ability, and validate her own instruction. Many friendships also evolve during these workshops, which provide a "networking" system that can prove invaluable to the serious dancer. Workshops also rent space to vendors who display their wares, allowing students who have limited access to dancewear and equipment a great opportunity to acquire all the necessities and keep up on trends.

GROUP OR PRIVATE INSTRUCTION?

Now it's time to talk about the different forms of instruction that you can choose from. Basically, you have two options — group instruction or private classes. As a rule, beginner students function best in a group situation and here's why.

One of the main skills that a novice dancer needs to learn is how to move within her own space and how to move in relation to others. The only way to define that space is to have peers to deal with. Dancing with others of similar age and ability also gives you a basis for comparison; a sense of competition, confidence, and humility; and a feeling of camaraderie. And it's just a lot more fun than dancing alone. Beginners are petrified of being singled out. They are well aware that they have a lot to learn and will make tons of mistakes, so they really feel more comfortable when there is safety in numbers. The only time I ever recommend one-on-one sessions for new students is if they have a particular physical problem that they would like help with, or if they need specific choreography or input pertaining to auditions or performance (i.e., an actor, a singer, or an athlete who needs help with movement).

The advanced or intermediate student can benefit from private instruction; however, it should always be balanced out with regular group classes. There will come a time when these more experienced students will need "fine tuning" or help undoing habitual mistakes. In these instances, private class can work miracles. Be advised that these sessions can be quite expensive, so be sure that they are necessary before signing up. Depending on the reputation and experience of the instructor or choreographer, they can cost anywhere from approximately ten dollars an hour to upwards of a hundred dollars an hour.

LENGTH OF THE CLASS

Aside from the form of your dance session, the class length should also be a consideration. I firmly believe that all dance classes should last a minimum of one hour (with the exception of creative movement for preschool children) and that each should concentrate on only *one* form of dance. It has been my experience that you need at least sixty minutes to get in a good warmup, combinations, corrections, and instructions, and any teacher who says that he can do it all in less time is not being realistic or doing a thorough job.

What is even less productive than short sessions is "combination classes." You will find that many studios and recreation centers (especially those that cater to very young children) try to sell parents on classes that combine two or more types of dance (a tap/ballet class, tap/tumbling/ballet, tap/jazz, etc.). They say that it's a great way to expose the children to multiple dance styles, when in reality, it makes the child confused (quantity versus quality). The class is almost totally unproductive, and it serves to put more money into the dance studio or center. More dance styles mean more dance shoes (a great plus for the studio that sells dancewear) and additional costumes (one for each kind of dance) at recital time. These sessions may serve to introduce a student to a variety of dance styles, but they really are not conducive to good solid dance training and won't give you the most dance instruction for your hard-earned dollar. You will discover as you read on that each form of dance has its own specialized warmup, music, content, feel, and attire. You just can't cram two or three types of dance into a half hour or an hour session and expect to get any comprehensive training or real results. My advice is to stick with the specialized classes and concentrate on one type of dance at a time.

THE TEACHER'S GENDER

Here is one more thing to consider — the sex of the teacher. Many parents have asked me if one is more preferable than the other. For the most part, the gender of the instructor is irrelevant. I must say, however, that I really believe boys and men should have a strong male role model as a teacher for a good portion of their training. This is not to say that a female can't give a boy excellent training. Many female instructors have extensive backgrounds in male physiology, have very strong styles, and possess the ability to choreograph for men and boys. But if you can find an equally gifted male dance instructor, I think he will make a major contribution to your own or your son's education. After all, it really does take one to know one!

WRAP-UP

Here it all is in a nutshell. Decide …

- ❏ whether you want private or group instruction
- ❏ what you can afford to pay for classes
- ❏ what extras you are willing to pay for (recitals, competitions, etc.)
- ❏ what level and quality of instruction you need
- ❏ if you have a preference for a male or female instructor

Find which type of facility offers what you want and start your search for the perfect class and teacher. No matter where you decide to start your dance experience, you will find that the journey will be a safe and happy one if you take along the right mental equipment to help you discover this wonderful new world. Follow this guidebook and have a great trip!

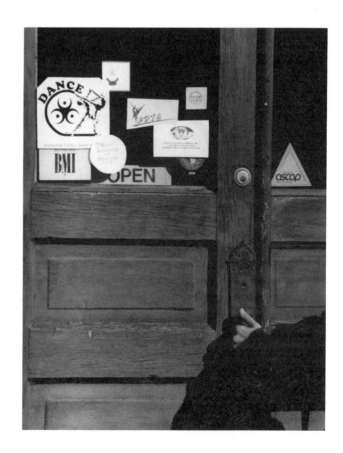

2
Licensing and Organizations

Certificate: A document providing evidence of status or qualifications, as one attesting to the completion of a course or the truth of facts stated.
Webster's Dictionary

Anyone can open a dance studio. All you need is a business license, a little money for advertising, music, and a space. You don't need to know how to dance or teach. You just need to convince the public that you do. Scary isn't it?

One of the ways that teachers try to validate themselves is by joining one of the many existing dance teacher organizations. They display their stickers on their studio door and believe that John Q. Public will automatically trust their teaching credentials because of their membership in these associations. Unfortunately, that is usually the case.

WHAT ASSOCIATION MEMBERSHIP DOES AND DOES NOT MEAN

Membership in any organization does not make a person a good dance teacher! It may furnish instructors and their students with some outlets and supplementary material, but membership in the majority of these groups does not in any way certify that its members are dance instructors who are knowledgeable in physiology, kinesiology, performance skills, theater, professionalism, or the real world of the working dancer. I am not saying that some organizations don't come darn close, but don't assume that a teacher's association with a particular organization means instant accreditation. Organizations only enhance a teacher's skills, and membership in these associations is certainly not mandatory. Many, many instructors are brilliant educators without their assistance.

As in everything, there are good apples and there are bad. In the case of dance organizations, the difference in quality is staggering. Some associations provide exemplary materials or teach excellent skills; others provide very limited actual benefits to students. Many groups are nothing more than teacher networking systems, which, after only minimal examinations, provide the teachers with fancy plaques, a "certification sticker" for the door, a "code of ethics," reduced insurance rates, a monthly newsletter, reduced tuition to their group's dance workshops and conventions (usually attended by the teachers to obtain recital choreography), and the right to enter students in yearly dance competitions.

Others are topnotch and concentrate on the process (actual teaching) of dance as opposed to the product (the routines and recital pieces) or the ins and outs of running a studio. In fact, certain renowned ballet associations have even developed syllabi (actual graded methods of teaching ballet) to provide a cumulative, safe foundation of instruction. Teachers are required not only to teach their students in a "tested" succession, but also to be tested and reevaluated themselves on a regular basis. For example, registered teachers of The Royal Academy of Dancing (R.A.D.), the oldest and largest ballet organization in the world, have to be retested every four years to keep up their certification and to be allowed to present their students for examinations. This is rare. In most cases it takes very little to join an organization. You take a little "exam," continue to pay your dues, and you're "in for life." No further testing (and I use the term loosely) is required. In actuality, many teachers who are displaying certain dance organization emblems took their "exams" ten, twenty, thirty, or even forty years ago and haven't been updated since.

Belonging to an organization is not necessarily an indication of a quality teacher or studio. Quality has to be assessed on an individual basis. It is true that the participating studio has access to a certain organization's benefits and materials, which may be important to you depending on your own needs and goals, but it may not mean much as far as actual teaching aptitude goes.

Keeping that in mind, I am going to provide you with the following information for evaluation purposes only. I am not going to be judge or jury. As an intelligent consumer, you will be able to read between the lines. Remember, you are looking for a qualified, educated, safe dance instructor.

MAJOR ORGANIZATIONS

The following are the major organizations that you may run into; however, there are numerous smaller groups that you could encounter, and many more are springing up all the time. Always dissect the *membership requirements* to determine whether or not association with a particular group adds to a teacher's qualifications. Networking helps everyone to be better at his or her craft, but beware of the teacher who claims that his membership in an organization "makes him qualified." Unless the standards and testing methods of an association are unquestionable, this claim is ludicrous.

The following information was copied verbatim from each organization's printed material, which they were gracious enough to provide to me for use in this chapter. Their objectives and goals are therefore their own and in no way express my opinions or my endorsement.

American Council on Exercise (A.C.E.)

"The exams test the knowledge essential to provide safe and effective exercise instruction to average, healthy people and handle typical questions and problems during exercise. They are not designed to qualify instructors as specialists for highly trained athletes, pre/postnatal women, older students, the physically handicapped, the morbidly obese, or people with known coronary heart disease or other physical limitations. However, certified instructors should have a basic understanding in these areas. Once you pass the A.C.E. Exam, you must renew your certification every two years."

TEST PREREQUISITES

1. Must be 18 years or older.
2. Must have current CPR certification.
3. Testing (3½ hour exam)

Certificates available include Aerobics, Personal Trainer.

Canadian Dance Teachers Association (CDTA)

"A national body whose aims are to establish and maintain, throughout Canada, a formal nonprofit organization of qualified dance teachers in all dance disciplines.

"To become a member (Ontario Branch): a teacher must take a qualifying examination, consisting of Theory, Demonstration, and Teaching segments.

"Classifications—Affiliate, Associate Member, Member, Fellow, and Patron. (Affiliates and Patrons cannot vote, hold office, or advertise as members of the CDTA.)"

The Cecchetti Council of America

"An organization dedicated to maintaining the standards and methods of ballet training established by Cav. Enrico Cecchetti. The organization uses his teaching and writings in a sequence of grades, carefully measured as to the degree of difficulty and physical development, and provides a system of accredited examinations to test the student's proficiency within those grades."

REQUIREMENTS FOR MEMBERSHIP

"Qualifications:

1. At least three years experience in teaching ballet.
2. Study and coaching with a qualified teacher of the method and sponsorship by a member.
3. Successful completion of at least one teacher's examination."
   Classifications include full members, associate, artistic, honorary, Junior branch.

Country Dance and Song Society (CDSS)

"An association of people with a common interest in English and American folk dance, music, and song. Among our members are recreational dancers, musicians, singers, teachers, callers, and dance historians dedicated to the enjoyment, preservation, study, and teaching of these rich traditions."

Types of memberships include contributor, individual, family, limited income, limited income family, subscriber.

Dance Educators of America (DEA)

"A National organization of qualified dance teachers who are accepted through a testing process."

REQUIREMENTS FOR MEMBERSHIP

"1. Each prospective Active member must successfully complete an examination in the form of dance he or she teaches.
2. Must be over 18.
3. Must have been teaching professionally for a minimum of three years, having had total responsibility in conducting his or her classes."

Offers Active membership; examinations in ballet, tap, jazz, acrobatics/gymnastics, and ballroom.

Dance Masters of America, Inc. (DMA)

DMA also has a Canadian chapter.
"The objects of Dance Masters of America are:

1. To advance the art of dance and improve the practice of teaching dance.
2. To enable dance teachers to meet for cooperative and collective study of conditions pertaining to their profession.
3. For the mutual interest and fraternal cooperation of its members.

REQUIREMENTS FOR MEMBERSHIP

"Membership is available to dance teachers — 18 years of age and over who have taught dance for a minimum of three years and who are actively engaged in the teaching of dance through ...

1. Ownership of a school
2. Operation of a school
3. Association with and/or assistantship to a qualified teacher
4. An institution of higher learning and pass membership examinations with a grade of at least 75%."

Imperial Society of Teachers of Dancing (ISTD)

"This society produces graduated syllabi in various branches of dancing and conducts examinations to test proficiency in them."

Exams offered include:

"Associate students aged 18 or upwards may enter the Associate exam to gain a teaching qualification status (AISTD) and professional registration.

"Associates may enter for the Licentiate (LISTD) exam when they have reached the age of 21 and completed three years of responsible teaching experience. Full registration is granted on completion of the practical exam and also written papers in Anatomy and Physiology and the History and Development of Western Dance.

"The Fellowship exam may be taken from the age of 25 after five years responsible teaching experience in the technique concerned.

"The Associate, Licentiate, and Fellowship examinations are all qualifications which are recognized and approved by the Council for Dance Education and Training."

(Pretty confusing to the layman, isn't it?)

International Teachers of Dance, Inc. (ITDI)

"Founded in 1984 and operating presently in the New Jersey area with members from Pennsylvania, Maryland, and Delaware (new chapters are being planned).

"To become a member, you must be at least 19 years of age and you must prove that you have taught for at least three years for a reputable dance school—studio, academy and present recommendation by your employer or director, also by members of ITDI, who know of your previous records."

National Dance Association (NDA)

National Dance Association is an Association of the American Alliance for Health, Physical Education, Recreation, and Dance.

"The National Dance Association is dedicated to promoting the development and implementation of sound philosophies and policies in all forms of dance and in dance education at all levels. By providing leadership for improvement in programs, materials and methods, NDA is active in identifying resources, and in gathering and disseminating pertinent information on dance to Association/Alliance members, other organizations, governmental bodies and agencies and to the general public. In cooperation with other arts and education organizations and structures in the Alliance, NDA strives to cultivate, facilitate, and promote the understanding and practice of dance.

"Membership in NDA includes dancers, choreographers, dance educators, therapists, dance science and medicine specialists, art administrators and Alliance members interested in dance."

Professional Dance Teachers Association, Inc. (PDTA)

"We are a Worldwide Organization of Dance Teachers, Choreographers, Artists, and Performers who have made their reputation in dance.

"Membership is available to all Dance Teachers who:

1. Are 18 years of age or older.
2. Have been teaching professionally for a minimum of two years, having had total responsibility in conducting his or her classes."

Types of membership are one-year, three-year, and five-year.

Registered Dance Therapist (D.T.R.)

According to the American Dance Therapy Association, D.T.R. is "... a registered dance therapist who has either a master's degree from a graduate program in dance therapy or a master's degree in a related field (i.e., dance, social work, psychology, counseling, or expressive art therapies)."

The Royal Academy of Dancing (R.A.D.)

"The R.A.D. is the largest, most influential public examining body for classical ballet throughout the entire world. The universally accepted gauge of dance teaching standards. The teacher examinations are based on practical experience and provide international recognition of the standards a teacher has attained. The Advanced Teacher's Certificate is the highest achievement a teacher can gain."

(Note: The types of membership and teacher registration available are diverse and, quite frankly, confusing to the lay person, so if you can't figure it out don't get discouraged. If the teacher in question is a member of the R.A.D., ask her exactly what type of membership and/or registration she has.)

"Registration available—Fully Registered (must be assessed every four years); Provisionally Registered." (Only Fully Registered or Provisionally Registered teachers may enter students for examinations. If you want yourself or your child to be examined, the teacher must be *Registered*.)

"Certificates available—Student Teaching Certificate, Teachers Certificate, Advanced Teachers Certificate."

There is no connection between membership of the Academy and Registration. You can be an R.A.D. member without being a Registered Teacher. I told you that this was all pretty confusing, didn't I?

Here are some titles that you might see after an R.A.D. teacher's name and what they represent:

A.R.A.D. — Associate of the Royal Academy of Dancing (Advanced Teachers Certificate) indicates the highest teaching qualifications. Can be given either for the teaching of Children or Major Syllabus.

L.R.A.D.—Licentiate of the Royal Academy of Dancing is awarded to students who have successfully completed the three-year teacher training course at the R.A.D. College.

F.R.A.D.—Fellowship of the Royal Academy of Dancing is an honor bestowed on an individual in acknowledgment of exceptional services to the academy.

OTHER RELEVANT AGENCIES

ASCAP, BMI, and SESAC, Inc.

The American Society of Composers, Authors and Publishers (ASCAP), Broadcast Music, Inc. (BMI), and SESAC, Inc. are music copyright regulatory agencies. Dance studios have to pay these organizations to use specific music during classes and in performance. These groups have nothing to do with dance itself!

AEA, SAG, AFTRA, AGVA

Actors' Equity Association (AEA), the Screen Actors Guild (SAG), the American Federation of Television and Radio Artists (AFTRA), and the American Guild of Variety Artists (AGVA) are unions you will find on résumés. Membership in one of the above generally means that the teacher has had some exposure to the paying professional world. Be careful, however, because there is a big difference between a person who has done two union TV commercials (which makes you a member of AFTRA and most likely has nothing to do with dance) and a person who has had a ten- or twenty-year *active* association with AEA or any or all of the above associations. Ask which shows, films, or credits she has, if she has acted *and* danced in these media, and if she is still active in the business and auditioning. (You don't want an actor as a dance instructor, unless of course she happens to be an expert in dance as well.)

WRAP-UP

There you have it. Do with it what you will. Remember, judge each teacher individually on her own merits, and try to determine how a teacher's membership in an organization makes her a better teacher and how it will benefit you or your child. Affiliation with a group or an organization *doesn't* make a teacher the right choice. It can be a determining factor, but it shouldn't be your only consideration. There is so much more. It doesn't matter how many initials a teacher has after her name, because ultimately it is her actions that will speak louder than words!

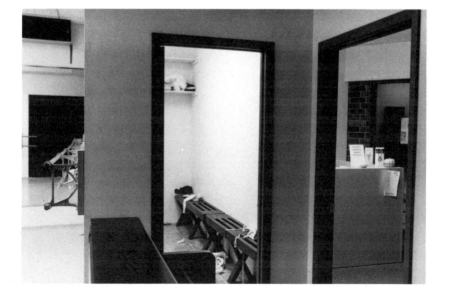

3
Basic Facility Requirements

All I ever needed was the music and the mirror ...
A <u>Chorus</u> <u>Line</u>

T he actual physical structure of the dance studio or facility doesn't really matter. Some of the best classes I ever took were in an old warehouse. The success of a class depends almost entirely on the teacher—not the surroundings. There are, however, a few specific things to look for and certain "tools" dance instructors use that need definition.

THE SPACE

A good dance facility consists of a clean, open space that has no obstructions and is equipped with changing areas, rest rooms, ventilation, a safe floor, some type of musical accompaniment, mirrors, and barres. It may not seem like much, but every detail is important. The space itself must be adequate in size and should be big enough to accommodate the number of students in the largest class. Dance, after all, is movement, and you cannot learn to move if you are constantly getting smashed in the face, banging into other students, bumping into poles, or hitting the ceiling. On the other hand, a tiny group of youngsters can feel really intimidated in a football field-size area, so the space should not be too large. A dance space should fit like a child's shoe. It should feel comfortable but have enough room to grow and wiggle your toes. The area should be free of pillars or supports, which could become dangerous when the moves speed up or the dancers start turning. It should be clean. Many dance moves involve sitting, lying, or rolling on the floor, and there is nothing more disgusting than becoming a human dust mop and picking up who knows what from a dirty floor!

Some type of ventilation should exist in the dance area, whether it is functional windows, which are ideal, or fans. Believe me, it only takes one fast-paced class to turn an entire studio into a smelly sauna, and a little fresh air can work wonders. If the classes are going to continue through the summer months, air conditioning might be another plus to look for, though most dancers prefer to sweat it out in fan-cooled studios rather than freeze in artificially cooled rooms.

There should be separate changing areas for males and females, and they should be distinct from the rest rooms. These rooms should also be reasonably neat (though dancers are known to be slobs), have a place to hang clothing, and be clean.

THE FLOOR

The floor is the big issue. The pertinent word here is CONCRETE. It's great for patios, roads, and statues of cherubs in the park but it's murder on the legs! *Never, never, never dance on concrete* or on a surface that has concrete directly underneath it. Continual dancing on these types of surfaces can take a dancer out of commission faster than you can say Rudolf Nureyev. Concrete has no "give" to it and will shock and jar muscles every time they come in contact with it. Before you know it, you could develop painful shin splints or lasting knee and back injuries. Find out how the floor is constructed. It is very easy to see if the floor is concrete, but it's impossible for the layman to tell just by looking at it whether the floor has a concrete base. You will have to ask.

The most desirable flooring is a wood floor that "floats" upon spacers, which are set in rows beneath it. It allows for flexibility on impact and is becoming more and more popular with the growth of the aerobic empire. This type of floor is extremely expensive, however, so you will not be likely to find it at a small neighborhood school. Many of these local businesses are located in "strip malls" or shopping centers and probably have linoleum or tile surfaces. If the surface has been laid on top of wood, then it is acceptable and, as long as it isn't slick, is relatively safe to dance on. Some owners of these types of studios who have been forced to "make do" with the existing flooring have purchased a roll-out hard rubber stage flooring that they use over the tile. This is also relatively common in studios where tap classes are minimal and where there is a new high quality wood floor in the dance area. The tap teacher rolls out the rubber floor during his classes to protect the more valuable floor underneath from the abuse of metal taps. The temporary surface is then rolled up and pushed out of the way when the class is over so that the other classes may use the wood floor. This type of surface is safe, but I find it a poor substitute for a good, broken-in hardwood floor.

MUSICAL ACCOMPANIMENT

After a safe floor, the next priority is good musical accompaniment. This can be either a clear, loud sound system (record player, cassette deck, or compact disc player); a piano with a full-time pianist; a drum and drummers or ethnic musicians; claves; or any combination of the above. Just be sure that some type of music or rhythm is used during classes and that it can be heard by *every* student, even over the thunder of twenty pairs of tapping feet.

Some studios have record players with variable speeds, so

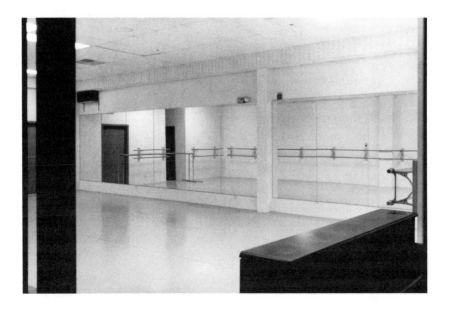

that the teacher can vary the rate of speed of a selection and adapt the music to the ability of the students. If you are a novice, this could be a plus. I find that when teaching beginners, these types of record players are an invaluable tool. A teacher does not have to waste a lot of precious class time looking through piles of records for one with the right tempo; instead she just turns the dial and the students keep on dancing. It really makes class move a lot more quickly. Record players, in general, tend to keep the classes hopping because they eliminate the need to "rewind," which can cause boring lulls in a session.

When it comes right down to it though, music is music. As long as there is some or a rhythmic equivalent, then it doesn't really matter what type is used. I do, however, have a real soft spot for live music. If you are interested in taking ballet and find a good studio with a pianist, or if a studio has live musicians, you are really fortunate. There is nothing as inspiring as the "real thing" when you're in class, and though it is not as common as it used to be, live accompaniment can still be found in many facilities. Drums or native instruments frequently add to the mood of modern, jazz, or ethnic classes and partaking in one of these sessions can be an exhilarating experience.

MIRRORS

Next on the list of necessities are mirrors. A person cannot know what she really look likes until she is faced with the reality of her own reflection. Mirrors are useful not only for comparison, but they also aid in spacing, teacher imitation, and mastering precision. They help the student develop peripheral vision, which is invaluable in performance (and can keep you from falling into the orchestra pit during a show). Mirrors also help keep a student's head up while dancing by allowing the student to follow the teacher's feet in the mirror instead of looking down as the steps are demonstrated. Keeping the focus up gives the dancers an overall view of the entire class and puts their movements into perspective, thus making class safer for all concerned. At least one wall of the studio should have an uninterrupted width of mirrors. The mirrors should be tall enough so that the dancers can see their entire bodies, and wide enough (in total width) so that all students can see in them at the same time.

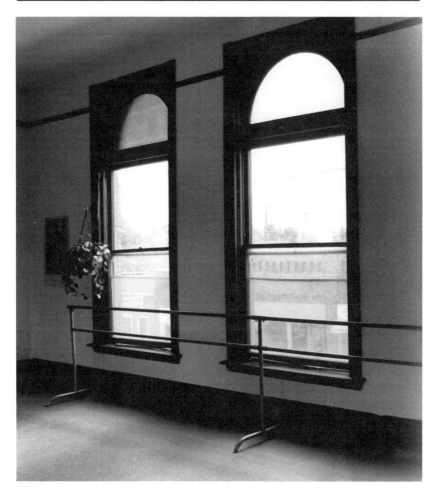

BARRE

A barre is the final essential element. It can be a wooden railing or metal pipe attached to a wall, a free-standing portable barre, or even the back of a chair (used in more advanced classes). Its function is support, and as long as the barre is stable, it will do the trick. If the school teaches all ages, barres of varying heights are necessary; however, most schools function adequately with only two levels. Depending on the school's curriculum, it may not be necessary to have barres at all. Some jazz, tap, and modern teachers are very successful without them, and there is no real need for them in ballroom and most ethnic classes. It is absolutely mandatory that ballet and pointe students have barres, so if you are signing up for either of these forms of dance, be sure that the studio is properly equipped or your training may be deficient.

WRAP-UP

Here is your checklist:

- ❑ Look for a clean, open, ventilated space with no obstructions.
- ❑ Be sure that the floor is safe.
- ❑ Check for changing rooms and adjacent rest rooms.
- ❑ Be sure that there is some form of musical accompaniment in class.
- ❑ Look for barres (if necessary) and mirrors.

If everything checks out, then you're in business. Maybe I should put it another way ... you have found a good business run by people who know what dancers need!

PART II

The Teacher

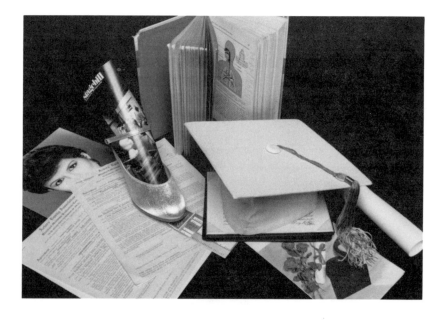

4
Credentials

How many people live on the reputation of the reputation
they might have made!
Oliver Wendell Holmes

OK! You have found a facility that looks and feels right, now how do you know if the teachers are qualified?

As shocking as it may seem, most people put more energy into researching the quality of their aerobic shoes than into checking out a prospective dance instructor or facility. They will let just about anyone twist, bend, or stretch their child or themselves without asking about the teacher's background, education, or credentials. Ask yourself this: Would you let a contractor who never studied construction, design, electrical wiring, or masonry build your house? Would you let a mechanic who doesn't know the parts of an engine tune up your car? For that matter, would you let someone whose background you haven't investigated or who had no previous experience baby-sit for your child? I don't think so! Why would you take dance classes from an instructor with few or no qualifications? The answer, of course, is that you shouldn't. Discovering whether a teacher is competent is not really all that difficult. You just have to ask the right questions and have enough knowledge to be able to interpret the answers.

USE YOUR POWERS OF OBSERVATION

Most of the investigative work involved in your quest for a good facility and dance instructor can be accomplished by being an astute observer. This is easy, and most people are generally comfortable assuming this role. It is when they have to step out of their "comfort zone," open their mouths, and ask questions that most consumers turn into babbling, insecure wimps. You suddenly feel as if you just "got off the boat" and landed in a foreign country where you don't speak the language. You are afraid of insulting the natives by saying the wrong thing. Though dance *is* a whole different world, if you arm yourself with some basic knowledge, you will be able to converse intelligently and get your questions answered. Remember, you are the customer. The studio is there to provide you with a service that you must pay for. You have every right to know what you are getting for your money! Don't be intimidated. People really love to talk about themselves, and if they feel threatened by your curiosity, they obviously have something to hide. Any qualified teacher will gladly tell you about his or her background, education, and teaching philosophies. If he has performed professionally, he can probably provide you with a copy of his résumé. Everything hinges on your approach. If you barge into the facility like the Ralph Nader of dance, be prepared to get tossed out on your rump. If you are friendly and act concerned and confident, however, you will get the results you desire.

TEACHING CREDENTIALS

In this chapter, I am going to talk about the different kinds of credentials and what's really important. Before I discuss these issues, however, I have to make a blanket statement. All the professional working experience and/or college education in the world *cannot* make a good teacher. This background can make someone who has been blessed with the gift of pedagogy a superb, safe, and highly qualified instructor. Today, it is not enough just to know a few steps, be a pleasant person, and have good business savvy in order to teach dance. Dance has developed into a demanding art form, and the physical and emotional damage that can be inflicted, especially in the very early stages of training, is staggering. It is absolutely mandatory that a teacher have some knowledge of both physiology and the real requirements — physical, mental, and emotional — needed to gain entry into the competitive world of the working professional. A college degree is not necessary and neither is a past

Broadway career. The knowledge can be obtained in a variety of ways — through reading, seminars, workshops, exposure to professionals, or any combination of the above. It is not important *how* the information is obtained, rather that the teacher recognizes the value of this knowledge and takes the steps to obtain it.

Right about now you're probably shouting, "Hold it! I just want to take class for fun!" That's all well and good because you are in the majority. Recreation, however, can quickly turn into a negative experience if you or your child sustains injuries under the tutelage of an uneducated instructor. *Granted, not everyone is going to dance upon the Great White Way, but that does not mean the quality of training a person receives should vary according to his or her aspirations.* Get your money's worth. You worked hard enough for it.

Outlined here are the very minimum qualifications that I believe a dance teacher should possess. Keep in mind that there are special qualifications you should look for depending on the type of dance you have chosen to study (see each individual chapter), but the following guidelines provide a basis for your assessment.

THE TEACHER'S QUALIFICATIONS

Teacher Training

Where did the teacher learn to dance? How long did he train? What did he take and from whom?

A dancer absorbs the knowledge and style of each mentor with whom he has studied. The more varied the prospective instructor's training, the more training he can pass along to his students. It is worse than presumptuous for any teacher to believe that his word is the "last word" in dance. A well-rounded instructor has an extensive background and has studied with many different people. He has also had many, many years of training. Beware of the teacher who says that he took dance classes as a child and "always dreamed" of opening a studio. If he only studied as a child, he could never possibly have progressed through the advanced levels, and his knowledge is probably outdated and very limited. I believe that every dance instructor must be at, or have attained at one time or another, an *advanced* level of expertise in the type of dance he or she is teaching.

Knowledge of Anatomy and Physiology

No one expects a dance instructor to be a doctor; however, a minimal understanding of the human body (large muscles, bones, joints, tendons, and pulse rates) plus treatment procedures of minor sport injuries (pulls, strains, basic first aid, etc.) is mandatory.

I have observed an interesting phenomenon among dancers. For the most part they are "klutzes." Put on the music and they turn into ethereal beings, but turn it off and they walk into walls. Like any other athletic endeavor, a certain number of bumps, bruises, aches, and pains are to be expected. Having a teacher who knows the inner body greatly minimizes the chance that more serious injuries will occur. Dancers also have special needs when it comes to warmup, and knowing the proper way to manipulate muscles to achieve the best performance is an invaluable skill.

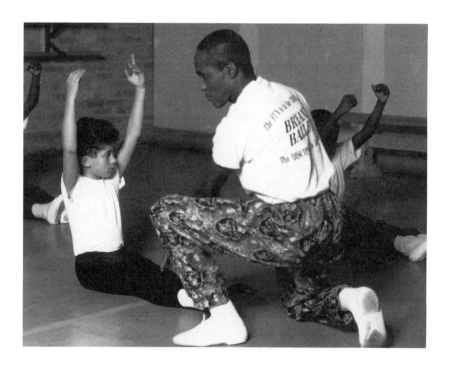

Think of a dance teacher as a sculptor. His job is to take a raw form and mold and work with it until it is something beautiful and has a life of its own. A sculptor cannot create without knowing the properties of the material he is working with, and a dance teacher cannot teach without knowing the limits and capabilities of his students' physiology.

Professional Performance Experience

If you have a serious desire to become a working dancer, your dance education must consist of more than physical training. I can't even begin to tell you about all the extra inside information that you will have to absorb along the way, but only one who has been there can give you a true insight into the world of the professional performer. However, a dance instructor with no personal performing experience can be just as effective in educating his students if he exposes them to working professionals. This can be done by attending workshops, having guest teachers, going to lectures, taking field trips, and providing constant exposure to dance programs and performances. As long as an instructor compensates for his own lack of personal stage experience, the students will receive a well-rounded dance education.

For the recreational student, having a teacher with a professional performance background is more a fascination than a real necessity, but this statement raises an interesting question. Are you absolutely sure that you or your child are only taking class for fun? What if you are really taking the first step toward a life-long, fulfilling career? The answer, of course, is that for the time being you really don't know. But wouldn't it be reassuring to know that you have received the very best in dance education just in case you do decide to follow the path to the footlights?

In deciding whether or not a performance background is an important asset in teacher selection, don't forget my initial statement. Having "field" experience is a plus, but it does not validate a person as a teacher. On the contrary, in many cases I have seen too much "professionalism" become a hindrance in a beginner class. A professional sometimes fails to realize the vast amount of knowledge that he or she has acquired and takes for granted. Subsequently, in a beginner teaching situation, he may find it difficult and frustrating breaking down steps to a level that the novice student can comprehend.

I have known many colleagues who find it impossible and unrewarding and who would rather wait tables than teach beginner dance in between shows or after retirement. Also, beginner students have never been exposed to the professional dance code of behavior and most possess few or no performance skills. The teacher who has constantly had to function at 150% in these areas, and who has become something of a purist, may find this exasperating and expect too much too soon. It takes a great deal of patience to teach "this is your right foot, this is your left," and not everyone is cut out for the task. If you are lucky enough to find a qualified instructor who has both patience and a solid performance background, then you will be twice blessed.

Continuing Study

Does the teacher still study and keep abreast of news, trends, and changes in style? Does he or she think it is important to keep growing in and learning about the field of dance— just as important for the teacher as it is for the student?

Nothing good grows in stagnant water. The art of dance is an ever-changing form of expression and, as with any art, its beauty can develop and grow only when it is fed and nurtured by the free-flowing waters of progress. It is a teacher's responsibility to keep his students stimulated and informed. This can only be accomplished if the instructor's knowledge is constantly expanded and his senses challenged.

When you walk into a studio or facility, look for dance and theater periodicals, books, workshop brochures, current performance programs, audition notices, etc. Ask the teachers if they still take class themselves or if they attend teacher seminars. Most teachers nowadays recognize the need to keep their choreographic material current, but not all realize that there is much more to dance than flashy recitals. If you can't get an assurance that the teacher is actively involved in today's dance world, then you would probably be better off looking somewhere else for instruction.

WRAP-UP

If a prospective dance instructor:

- ❏ has had varied and extensive training,
- ❏ has a basic working knowledge of physiology,
- ❏ performed professionally or exposes his students to professionals,
- ❏ has continued his own dance training and education by taking class and/or keeping abreast of dance trends and news, then ...
  his credentials are A-plus. Give yourself the same grade for doing your homework.

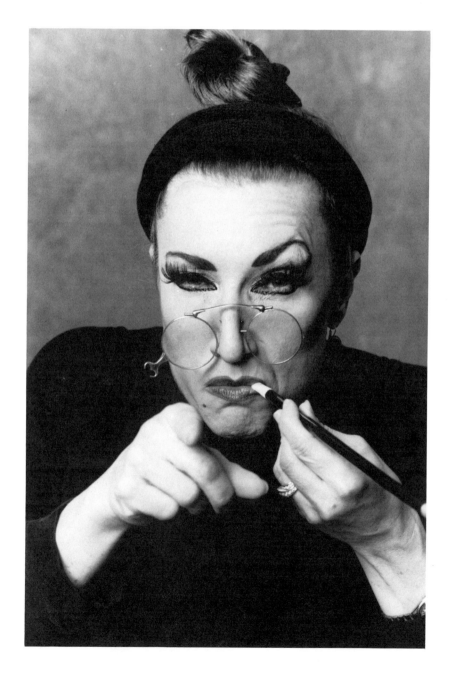

5
Personality

Let's face it—dance is fun! No matter what your reasons are for "joining the dance," underneath there is the simple fact that it really gives you a terrific high. Granted, it is a discipline and to master it requires endless hours of repetitive training, but it doesn't have to be boring or monotonous. On the contrary, dance class should be a joyous adventure, and a student should look forward to class with happy anticipation. Not every day is going to be a holiday, but an enthusiastic, patient, supportive, and prepared teacher can keep the morale at a pretty consistently high level and be a real and lasting source of inspiration.

To screen a prospective teacher to see if she possesses these qualities, it is necessary to watch the instructor teach an actual class. Most studios have no problem with observers, and some encourage it on a limited basis. Once inside, you need to know what to look for. This is really quite simple, and you should be able to form an opinion relatively quickly.

ENTHUSIASM IS CONTAGIOUS!

Enthusiasm is absolutely mandatory, especially in the early stages of instruction. There is nothing worse than walking into a dance class where the instructor is obviously bored silly and would rather be undergoing major surgery than teaching dance. A real pedagogue doesn't view teaching as merely a job. To her it is a labor of love and a serious commitment. Yes, it is true that it is extremely difficult to be "up" all the time, but it goes with the territory. Enthusiasm is contagious! It helps strip away the inhibitions that students bring with them into class, and it relieves the everyday tension that permeates our lives, thus freeing up the students to learn. Loving what you do and passing along that love and dedication to other people, especially impressionable beginners, is a true talent.

It is amazing how much influence a teacher can have on novice students, especially if they are young children. It is my belief that teachers who, hour after hour, day after day, week after week, work with rooms full of starstruck, fidgety, and sometimes less than enthusiastic youngsters should receive halos and be canonized. Let's be realistic. The little devils and their normal energetic behavior have a tendency to get on your nerves! A person must either be nuts or *really* love kids—a lot. Not everyone does, and if you are lucky enough to find someone who is a great teacher and a cross between Captain Kangaroo and Alice on "The Brady Bunch," then sign up your little darling and consider yourself fortunate.

IMPORTANT CHARACTER TRAITS

Along with an undying enthusiasm and the patience of Job, there are other character traits that a good teacher of beginners should possess. Tact and sensitivity are certainly high on the list. A teacher must have the ability to give *constructive* criticism and do so selectively and kindly.

When you observe the instructor in question, ask yourself these things. Does the teacher give corrections and make adjustments or is she just dancing for herself and going through the motions? Are the corrections given in both a general manner and on an individual basis, and are they given constructively? Watch out for teachers who "browbeat" their beginning and intermediate students. Novice students need tender love and care, encouragement and direction, and there is plenty of time later on, in the more advanced stages, to bring the realities of the demanding dance world into clearer focus.

Also be wary of an instructor who constantly "picks on" a particular pupil. There will always be personality conflicts and students with lesser potential; however, it is these people who benefit the most from guidance and understanding. Students who are "different" or who have handicaps or learning disabilities need a teacher whose patience and devotion are beyond question. These special dancers place additional demands on instructors, and great care should be taken to place them in an environment where they can grow and learn without humiliation or alienation. If you or your child fall into this category, you must find a teacher who realizes that encouragement can work miracles. Conversely, watch out for favoritism. It is one thing to use a particular student as an example, but if this student and his or her "superior ability" are constantly being referred to or used to embarrass the rest of the class, then feelings of resentment and jealousy will fester and turn an otherwise delightful class into a nightmare.

PROFESSIONALISM

Professionalism is the next thing to look for. Dance is learned by imitation—whether it be by copying a teacher's steps or style or by following the example that an instructor sets as to behavior and accepted modes of conduct. A teacher should be properly attired in dancewear and dance shoes, be in reasonably good physical condition, and not condone or partake of injurious habits (smoking, taking drugs, etc.) or validate unprofessional behavior in class (gum chewing, eating, etc.). A student who is looking to her instructor as a role model will think these actions acceptable and possibly set her own standards accordingly. Bad habits are hard to break!

PUNCTUALITY

Being on time for class is another way in which a teacher can show self-discipline and a respect for her art. Nothing aggravates me more as a busy consumer than my time and money being wasted. If I pay for an hour class and it's supposed to start at 8:00, then I should get an hour class, and it should not begin at 8:15 or 8:30. One of the considerations when choosing a particular class may be the convenient way that it fits into your own particular schedule. The *least* that a teacher can do is be punctual. Barring acts of God, this really shouldn't be difficult.

After all, the teacher is being paid for a specific block of time, and the students all managed to get to class on time, so it really is not too much to ask that she make it there, too.

PREPARATION

Teachers are also paid to be prepared. Musical selections and dance combinations should be found and worked out before-hand, and students should not have to stand around wasting valuable class time letting their warmed up muscles get cold while a teacher tries all the selections in a stack of records or dances in front of the mirror for an eternity trying to come up with a new step. Some of the best choreography does happen in-stantaneously, but most dance instructors aren't brilliant "on the spot" choreographers, and some pre-class preparation is usually needed to come up with something appropriate and innovative.

Watch the class. It should flow. If it doesn't, and there seems to be an awful lot of "dead time" when no actual dancing, demon-stration, or verbal instruction occurs, then ten to one, the teacher isn't prepared.

During your surveillance, also watch to see if the teacher has control. Chaos is not conducive to learning, and a little firmness is essential when dealing with large groups, young children, or dancers wearing noisy tap shoes. Gestapo techniques, however, are unnecessary, and there are a lot easier ways to maintain or-der and achieve the desired effects. Preparedness is really the key. If the students are constantly moving and their minds aren't allowed to wander, the class will be more productive and enjoyable.

WRAP-UP

If the teacher has respect for her art, herself, and her students, you will be able to see it, and in turn, the students will radiate respect for their instructor, listen attentively to her words of wisdom, and feel fortunate to have her as their mentor and friend. You will, too!

PART III

The Kinds of Dance

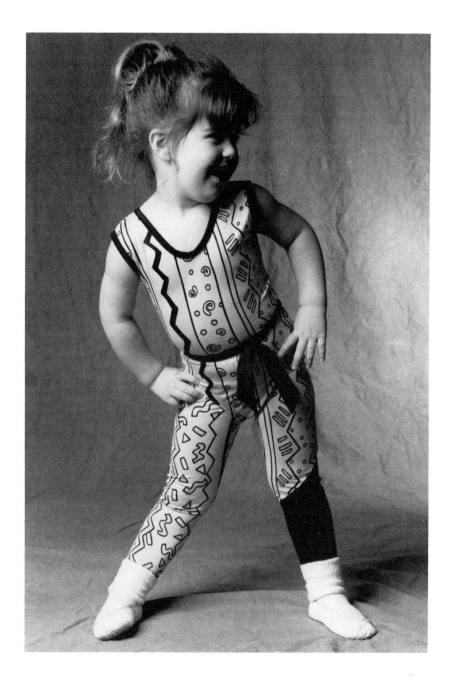

6
Predance

WHAT'S THE RUSH?

Everywhere you look today, you see businesses and classes that cater to kids. From computer classes to cooking classes, they are all there for the taking. The dance business is no exception. In fact, it seems to be a major contributor to this trend. Most of the studio's revenue, and a good percentage of the profits that are made by recreation centers, come from dance sessions for children. In many, many cases, these sessions are for those of preschool age, and it has even become the "thing to do" for parents to stand in line and shell out big bucks to give little Sally or Johnny every opportunity in life before they are old enough to go to academic school. It's quite an interesting phenomenon!

I happen to have pretty strong opinions on these types of dance classes, but before I get onto the soap box, let's get a little more specific as to what the term "predance" really means. Classes that fall into this category can take a variety of forms. To simplify things, I am going to separate the term "predance" into two classifications. The first includes classes claiming to teach or introduce some specific form of dance. They are usually called Pre Ballet, Pre Tap, Baby Ballet, Baby Tap, or something cute like Dancing Dolls or Tiny Tappers. For the sake of discussion, we will call these "predance." The second type includes all of the preschool "creative movement" classes that don't stress a particular dance style but concentrate more on movement exploration.

THE HAZARDS OF PREDANCE

Now it's time for me to step onto the platform and have my say. Hold onto your hats! Let's start with predance—my pet peeve. These are the sessions where adorable (barely potty-trained), chubby little tots don equally adorable expensive dancewear and run around learning the likes of "I'm a Little Teapot." I have a serious problem with these classes when they are sold to the public as a necessity to "prepare" little ones for participation in regular classes or as the first step toward a budding career. Baloney! Parents, listen up: these classes are, except for their entertainment value, total wastes of time and money! They can, in some cases, even be detrimental to your child. I know that there are loads of Park & Recreation instructors and dance teachers out there who would like to string me up by my toe shoe ribbons (and who stand to lose a lot of revenue) because I am taking this stand, but believe me, my statement is based on fact.

Teaching tiny preschool children dance positions, stretches, terms, and routines *will not* and I repeat *will not* accelerate a child's dance career. It will keep the kids amused for half an hour or so, and it will cost you anywhere from a few dollars a class to hundreds of dollars (if you get caught up in recitals). But there is no need to preempt regular dance classes with this type of "instruction." As a consumer, the trick is to know what you are really getting for your time and money and what you are not. You notice that I say "you" and not "what your child wants." Let's face it. At three to six years old, they really don't know. What they do know is that they (like all children) love music, movement, and pretty costumes. That's great, but they don't know how to direct their energies, so it is your job to be their guide.

As a parent myself, I know how very difficult it is to say NO to your kids, and I have sure made (and continue to make) my share of mistakes. At certain times, however, especially when one of mine starts begging for something or to do something, I am reminded of words of wisdom I once heard. "Children should be given what they *need* not what they *want*." In the case of dance lessons, a teary-eyed four year old might be pleading to take ballet, but it's the wise parent who knows that she doesn't *need* to for another three or four years.

So, if you are looking to have your child actually learn a specific type of dance, then my advice would be to put that precious leotard (the one with the attached tutu and rhinestones) back on the rack, put your checkbook back in your pocket, and wait until your child's body and maturity are really ready. If you want her to run around, bounce, and play then go ahead and sign her up. Remember, however, that she can do the same things at home (for free) and that enrollment in this glorified day care will not further her theatrical career. It could, in fact, if taught by a boring, uneducated instructor, cause her to withdraw and dislike dance altogether.

Kids Under Pressure

Over the last twenty years or so, I have noticed an interesting but potentially dangerous trend developing. Many, many parents, for whatever reasons, seem to be compelled to drown their very, very young children in a sea of useless activities. Before children have even entered full-time school, and before they can absorb the onslaught of information or completely benefit from the experience, parents are enrolling them in everything from Baby Pom Pom, gymnastics, and T-ball to competitive sports or dance classes. As I said, in some cases, depending on the instructor or number of classes taken at one time, it could lead to serious physical, emotional, and developmental problems. I have seen well-meaning parents taxi their tiny children to and from a studio two to three times a week to participate in a variety of predance classes. And more often than not, these children are signed up for other activities/classes as well. The parents are run ragged, the children are exhausted and confused, and everyone has lost sight of the initial objective—FUN! There seems to be no time left in their busy little schedules for them just to be kids. Some may as well have their own appointment books!

What's the hurry? Is there really a *need* to expose a child to activities or dance so quickly? I honestly don't think so. I started tap at age five, and it didn't really make a difference in my career. Looking back, I wish my mom had waited and started my dance education with solid ballet training. I have worked with many brilliant dancers who began their instruction late in life (some as late as college), and I have also known many people who would have had a chance at a serious dance career had they not lost the love of dance at an early age under the "guidance" (or lack thereof) of an overenthusiastic parent.

Little children are not supposed to have pressure in their lives. They should not be required to practice, memorize, or perform when all they really want to do is respond naturally to the music. Put on a tape and let them play dress-up at home. Believe me, there will be plenty of time for them to learn the specifics of dance later on. Why not invest the money and time in trips to the local library, zoo, or children's museum to learn about and study movement? In the long run, everyone will be better off.

As difficult as it may be to wait until your child is of the appropriate age to begin legitimate dance instruction (see each individual chapter for guidelines), it can be the smartest thing for both your child and your bank account. You will quickly discover that the "skills" they would have been taught in years of predance classes will be learned in the first few weeks or so of regular dance instruction *when begun at the right age*.

There is an even bigger plus. Their minds and bodies are ready for the instruction and they will (1) be at less risk of physical and psychological damage; (2) be able to retain the information; (3) enjoy the lessons on an emotional level; and (4) not be burnt out by having been subjected to the rigors of unnecessary weekly classes for the last two to four years. The bottom line is that by simply waiting a few years, your child will be physically, mentally, and emotionally prepared to *really* learn to dance. You will save yourself a lot of time and energy and enough money to give your child first class instruction.

CREATIVE MOVEMENT

All right, enough said. Now on to creative movement. If you are intent on giving your little one a group movement experience, a good creative movement class would be your best bet. This type of session, *if* taught by a qualified dance educator (especially one whose base is modern dance), can be safe, educational, and fun. The problems lie in finding a bona fide creative movement class. The term "creative movement" has became a catchall phrase for "baby dance classes," so you will need to understand what the teacher should be trying to accomplish to be sure that you have found the real thing.

Rhythm, timing, space and its use, levels, directions, and size are the main focus in class, and each child and his or her body (and its use) should be considered unique. The objective is for the students to go on an individual internal exploration to discover their own movement and its relation to others. There should be no pressure, practice, memorization, or rights or wrongs—only the pure enjoyment of the movement itself. Basically, creative movement is as free as the child.

In searching for a good class, you might begin with your local university. Modern dance is usually the forte of their dance departments, and "Creative Movement for Children" (or some such course) is usually a requirement of dance majors. Classes for children will sometimes be offered to the public (usually on Saturdays), so that the student teachers can work with actual kids (under the supervision of a professor or department head). If you can find one of these classes, sign up with confidence.

If you strike out on the college level or you don't have a university nearby, look to a dance studio or company that specializes in modern dance or that falls under the heading of a "Professional School" (see Chapter 1). No matter where you find a class, try to observe an actual class in action before you sign up. Check that the class has the right focus (as described above) and that it is taught by a qualified, experienced, friendly adult instructor who understands the complexities of dance and who *really* likes children.

You will notice that I specified *adult* as one of the teacher requirements. I did that for a very specific reason. There are many studios that think of the baby classes as merely extra income, don't take them seriously, and let their older (and usually inexperienced) teenage students (many times the owner's son or daughter) teach these classes. Though, nine times out of ten, these teens are cute and personable, they are not really equipped to give a complete movement experience. Look for an adult who has a solid background and interest in dance education for the very young, and I think you will get the best results.

WRAP-UP

If you are intent upon putting your three- to five-year-old child in dance, remember that a predance class:

❏ *will not* accelerate a child's dance education,
❏ is only for enjoyment,
❏ could, if taught by an inexperienced teacher, do more harm than good.

A *real* creative movement class, however, taught by a qualified, experienced, friendly adult instructor can help a young child take her first steps toward a lifelong love of dance.

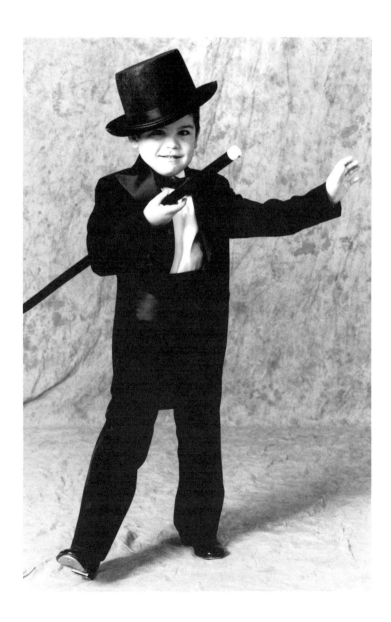

7
Tap Your Troubles Away

> *Got a little rhythm, a little rhythm*
> *A rhythm that pit-a-pats through my brain ...*
> George and Ira Gershwin, "Fascinating Rhythm"

When I die, I want to be buried with my tap shoes on. The pall bearers will be dressed in sequins, and I will have on white tails, high cut trunks, and fishnet stockings. I want to be ready to dance UP (a great assumption on my part) that long staircase to the pearly gates, just as Shirley Temple and Bill Robinson tapped up the stairs in *The Little Colonel*.

I tap everywhere! I have publicly embarrassed nearly every member of my family by beating out a rhythm with my feet in an inappropriate place and have been known to click my way down the aisles of the supermarket, across streets, and even behind the wheel of my car (which neither I nor my insurance agent really recommend). My great-grandfather on my mother's side was an Irishman who loved to clog and my father's ancestors wore noisy wooden shoes and rejoiced in the crisp sounds that they made during their daily trek down the tulip-lined cobbled streets of their homeland. I am proud to have carried on the family tradition.

THE JOYS OF TAP

Tap is a great way to learn about rhythm, gain confidence, relieve stress, firm up those "gams," and just have a terrific time. If you are looking for a fun recreational activity for yourself or your child, then tap is tops. If you are pursuing a serious dance career in today's market, tap is a necessity.

Tap does have its negative side. People who tap have been known to experience recurring dreams of becoming Ann Miller or Gene Kelly, and tap dancing is definitely addictive. If those hazards don't bother you, then make a beeline to the nearest dance studio and be prepared to find heaven!

MINIMAL PHYSICAL RISKS

Unlike ballet, the physical risks that could be encountered in tap dancing are minimal if not almost nonexistent. Training can begin at almost any age. If a child is mature enough to practice self-control, pay attention consistently for an hour, and function constructively in a group situation (I recommend age seven or eight), then they can start to tap. It is also a terrific way to get boys interested in dance. Some of the famous movie musical role models (Gene Kelly, Fred Astaire, Donald O'Connor, Danny Kaye, etc.) have given tap its dignity and have made it not only acceptable but desirable for males to learn. In fact, thanks to them and their talents, tap dancing has really risen to a physically demanding art form.

In the early stages, tap doesn't require a tremendous amount of physical strength or stamina so the average adult or senior citizen with repressed Rogers or Astaire fantasies can sign up for classes with confidence. But don't be fooled. Even though tap dancing is relatively safe, you should be just as careful in your selection of a teacher and facility as you would with any other form of dance.

LEARNING TO TAP

A good beginner tap teacher must have the patience of a saint, the sense of humor of a standup comedian, and the talents of a drill sergeant. His job is to walk boldly into a room jammed full of untrained, overenthusiastic, nervous students who are "armed" with potentially irritating metal devices attached to their shiny new shoes, and to mold them into a precision rhythm group. It's a painstaking process for the instructor, while the students, who are enthralled with the pleasant discovery that their feet can make sounds, are having an absolutely ethereal experience. Students generally get so excited about their revelation that they try to run before they can walk, and the teacher must pull back firmly on the reins to avoid a stampede.

Learning to tap is very similar to learning to read. You must build a firm foundation of the basics and a knowledge of the way each step sounds in order to progress to a level of expertise. If a teacher does not dissect each step as it is presented, and if students aren't taught *slowly* and in the correct sequence, you could find that as time goes on and as the music and combinations speed up and get more complex, your ability to comprehend could come to a screeching halt. A tap teacher must have a great personality, but it must be balanced by a gentle firmness and knowledge of the teaching process.

Since you have never tapped, determining whether an instructor possesses this knowledge is hard. However, observation is the key. Watch the class in which you wish to enroll or one that is of the same level and taught by the same instructor. Any dance establishment worth its salt will not only allow this but encourage it. If there are no classes in session when you wish to enroll, check out the qualifications of the studio or facility and the credentials of the teacher in question (see Chapters 2 and 3) and make an evaluation after you have actually taken a few classes. No matter when you make your observation, there are a few basic things to watch for in a class.

DRESS

A competent teacher should require dancewear. The whole body is used in dance, not just the feet. A good beginner tap teacher must be able to monitor weight placement and posture and should introduce the proper use of arms for balance, line, and style. Since tap dancing comes from the body's "hinges," the legs should be clearly defined so the teacher can see if the movements have their origins in the hip sockets, knees, or ankles. Watch out for "street clothes" in class! Leotards and tights are the proper uniform and give the necessary torso and leg visibility while allowing for freedom of movement. The color and style of the basic leotard and tights dance uniform really doesn't matter much in tap class unless the studio has a specific dress code or preference. Short tap skirts and tap pants (very short shorts) have become the norm; however, sweat pants, loose-fitting shirts, and bulky leg warmers should be avoided. Boys and men should wear comfortable tapered pants that allow movement or "jazz pants" (a tight-fitting knit pant designed for dance). A snug fitting T-shirt should be worn on top. Tights for males are also acceptable when worn over a leotard, and don't forget the importance of an athletic supporter or a dance belt (a supporter that is sleeker and was designed to be less obvious under dancewear) for safety's sake.

THE RIGHT SHOES

Watch out for "high-heeled" tap shoes on females in a beginner class. This is of the utmost importance. There are basically two types of tap shoes for girls and women: (1) flat shoes either of a patent or leather tie type or a flat "jazz shoe," which resembles a leather tennis shoe; or (2) leather shoes with instep or ankle straps, which have tapered heels ranging in height from 1 to 3 inches.

Almost all tap technique comes from developing the use of the ankles, stretching the Achilles tendon (the large tendon that runs from the heel up the back of the calf), and the flexing and pointing of the instep and toes. It takes years to be able to manipulate the feet properly to achieve the desired effects, and this cannot be accomplished by starting out in heels. Men are historically better tappers, and there is no doubt that it is due primarily to the fact that they always wear flat shoes and have developed better control of their balance and ankles.

You must train with your feet *flat* on the ground in order to grasp the concepts and ultimately gain the strength and expertise needed to accomplish the same steps while wearing a pair of high-heeled shoes. These shoes are very similar in concept to pointe shoes in ballet. They are only for the advanced student and should not be worn prematurely. I don't care how badly you yearn to look like a chorus girl, you will never make it as one unless you start at the beginning with FLAT shoes! A good instructor will guide you every step of the way (no pun intended) and will tell you when it is time to "rise to the occasion" and don your first pair of heels.

LOOK FOR A SAFE FLOOR

Because of the nature of tap and the constant abuse that the legs receive, the surface of the floor, and more important, the surface *beneath* the floor are of great importance. NEVER, NEVER, NEVER dance on concrete or on a floor that has concrete directly under it! Constant tapping on such a surface can quickly give you a nasty case of shin splints (a tearing of the muscle away from the front of the shin bone), which is extremely painful and debilitating. Wood, tile, or linoleum that has a subfloor of wood or materials that absorb shock (see Chapter 3 for specifics) are the most desirable surfaces. Don't be afraid to ask what the floor has underneath it! You or your child are the one at risk, and a responsible dance studio owner would not allow his or her facility to have dangerous flooring.

COUNTING AND USING TERMINOLOGY

The basis for tap is rhythm and timing. A student must be trained to count to the beat of the music and divide each count mentally into many pieces to form a rhythm or step. The counting of each step in class is absolutely necessary if the beginning student is to develop the timing that goes hand in hand with tap. If a teacher doesn't count in lower level classes, you can be pretty sure that he doesn't know the needs of his students.

Also listen for the use of tap terminology in instruction. Unlike other forms of dance in which the names of steps or groups of steps vary from teacher to teacher, most tap terms are the same everywhere. Knowledge of the names of the steps gives a dancer the extra edge of being able to execute combinations on verbal command rather than waiting to have them demonstrated (a real plus in auditions). If an instructor doesn't use the tap vernacular, he probably doesn't know it.

CONTROL OF THE CLASS

Enthusiasm runs rampant in tap class, and a great percentage of the time students unintentionally get caught up in the excitement of a new step or combination and go into what I fondly refer to as "tapper trance." People start internally trying to figure out the new challenge by themselves as soon as it is presented and forget that there are other students in the room. Everyone starts tapping at the same time but not together, and the noise level in the class gets way out of hand. If the students happen to be youngsters, there is the added problem of their natural lack of self-control. A teacher must be able to bring everyone back to the real world, restore order, and teach class in unison. Remember, you are paying for this time period and don't want to waste valuable class time listening to chaos. If there seems to be no control or organization, and everyone just seems to have "happy feet," this class will not give you your money's worth.

TAP SOUNDS

One other thing is worth mentioning. During your observations you might detect that the sounds of the taps vary from studio to studio. Don't let this confuse you. Though it will not become an issue until you actually sign up for instruction and have to purchase your shoes, it certainly is something that deserves clarification.

There are many different brands of taps, and the substance that they are made of (type of metal or wood), their design and shape, and the way that they are mounted (tight or loose) vary the quality of the sound you hear. The type of studio floor also is a factor in the overall tonal quality. No matter what, you should hear a *clarity* of sound.

Let's talk taps. There are two main types that you may encounter: (1) the standard solid plate (of which there are *many* variations) and (2) the "jingle" tap, which has a loose piece of metal in the center that wiggles as you dance. The latter is easily recognizable because you will hear the tap make a sound even when it is not touching the floor (i.e., when a person is walking or picking up his feet). It is all a matter of teacher preference as to the type of tap used in the studio, and very often the choice is left up to the student, but if you are a dance novice, you might need a little direction. I feel that the jingle tap hinders the beginning student's ability to hear the sounds clearly and to differentiate between the actual step and the jingle. As a teacher, I also find jingle taps distracting and unnecessary; however, some studios seem to like them.

What is of greater importance than the type of tap is the fit of the tap to the shoe. Since tap dancing has gained in popularity, many manufacturers of dance footwear have expanded their lines of tap shoes. With each new toe or heel design, a new tap has been created to fit the shoe's sole. The shape of men's shoes has not changed drastically, so the fit of their taps does not seem to be as much of a problem. Women, however, have many more types of shoes to choose from and subsequently a harder time choosing the right size of tap. Be sure, and I can't stress this enough, that your taps fit the *entire* toe and heel area of the shoe and extend all the way to the outer edges of the sole. A rubber "skid pad" should be glued to the ball of the shoe adjacent to the toe tap to keep slipping on slick surfaces to a minimum, and the place where the toe tap and skid pad meet *should be flush.*

All of the above can be done by any reputable shoe repair service, and a little grinding with a metal file at the base of the tap will get the right results. If these two surfaces are not the same thickness, you will feel as though you are dancing on a ridge, and balance will be difficult if not impossible. In order to tap efficiently, the bottom of a tap shoe should feel like any other comfortable shoe, and a dancer should not be able to feel the tap or pad on the bottom. Proper fitting of taps can make the difference between a secure, productive dancer and one who is unbalanced and frustrated.

WRAP-UP

Go observe a tap teacher and class in action and ask yourself these questions:

- ☐ Do the students dress properly?
- ☐ Are the beginner female students wearing *flat* tap shoes?
- ☐ Is the floor a safe surface for dance? (Don't be afraid to ask questions. NO CONCRETE!)
- ☐ Does the teacher count and use tap terminology?
- ☐ Does the teacher have patience, a sense of humor, and control of the students?

If you can answer YES to all of the above, put on your patent leathers and have a ball!

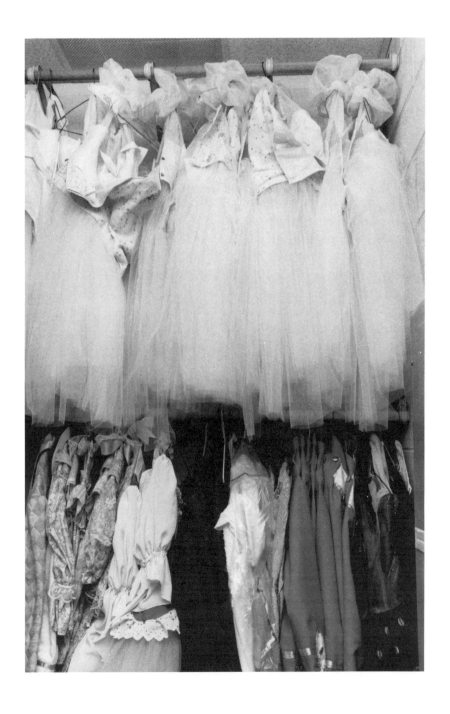

8
Visions of
Sugar Plum Fairies

Everything is beautiful at the ballet ...
A Chorus Line

Ah, ballet—the loftiest of the art forms! What child hasn't longed to wear tutus and satin slippers or be the Prince who leaps effortlessly across the stage? Whether you are fulfilling that child's dream or finally acting it out for yourself, exercise great care in your choice of teacher and facility. Ballet is probably the most abused dance form when it comes to qualified dance instruction. You need to call upon all of your resources to ensure that the training you or your child receive is administered by someone who really "knows her stuff" and, more important, is extremely knowledgeable in physiology.

"But my little girl just wants to run around in a leotard with her hands up over her head." Well, then my advice to you would be to buy her some rhinestone-studded dancewear and a cassette of *The Nutcracker* and let her have a field day—at home! Your other option is to enroll her in a creative movement class that has the freedom a preschooler needs, and where rhythmic games, counting, and coordination are stressed instead of ballet technique.

I wish I had a nickel for every time a mother came into one of my studios and proudly announced, "She's a natural! She walks around on her tiptoes *all by herself!*" You could literally feel my entire staff wince as the parent rattled on and on extolling the virtues of her little preschool star. I would gently take the prima ballerina's mom by the hand, give her a BIG cup of coffee, and lead her into my office to "discuss" her daughter's dancing future.

My coffee might have been hard to digest, but the truth was even harder to swallow. The reality of the situation, then and now, is that *almost all* preschool children dance on their tiptoes. They also bounce to the beat of the music. *It's their job!* It's the natural right of every little person under the age of five. This is not to say that somewhere down the line this little dumpling won't be the lead dancer in *Swan Lake*, but she has loads of time and tons of training to get through in the meantime. Let her enjoy the music for awhile without subjecting her to the regimen of ballet.

THE CASE AGAINST EARLY BALLET

All the professional dancers I interviewed agree that ballet—serious ballet—before the age of eight or so is totally meaningless except for the recreational and social benefits. They further concurred, and I quite agree, that it can be very harmful to young developing bodies if taught by someone who is trying to inflict *technique* on preschool-age children.

After that statement, I should probably barricade myself into a secure foxhole somewhere in anticipation of the barrage that will be forthcoming from dance studio owners everywhere. That, however, is to be expected. A dance studio's revenue depends heavily on the "kiddie" classes, and any question of their validity would come as a personal affront and threat to the owners' reputations. You see, as the children enter puberty and become intimidated by their bodies, enrollment and attendance usually falter. Also, the kids' involvement in other outside activities (cheerleading, sports, boys) sometimes pushes their desire to dance into the background. Thus most studios rely on the younger student for a great deal of their livelihood. I will even don a bulletproof vest, crawl deeper into the dirt, and say that, in my opinion (and again in the opinion of working dance professionals), the ballet "training" a child receives from age three to age seven could be taught in its entirety in a three-month period of instruction with a qualified teacher and retained by most eight year olds. Furthermore, the risk of bodily injury would be lessened considerably by simply waiting a few years to start ballet. Most eight-year-old children also possess the mental capabilities required to begin grasping the intricate concepts of ballet, whereas very young children have enough problems standing still or focusing for more than a matter of minutes.

Go ahead, teachers, and load your guns (I know that I'm going to get it with both barrels for this) because I'm going to really tell John Q. Public the facts.

At let's say $5 per class times 34 weeks of instruction (based on one class per week with the summer vacation off), that equals ballet tuition of $170 per year. Multiply that times 4 (instruction from ages three through seven) and you get $680. Add to that the cost of numerous leotards, tights, and ballet slippers ("Gee, she's growing like a weed!"), hair ribbons to match, little shiny plastic cases sporting ballet dancers to carry it

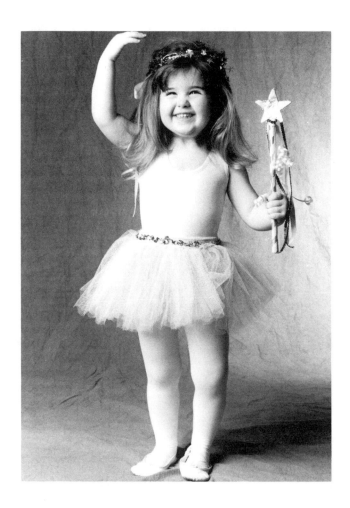

all in (a must), and recital costumes (we wouldn't want to waste all that talent by not showing it off), and you have probably dropped something in excess of $1,500. That's an awful lot to put out to have a budding preschool star enjoy herself. After you tack on transportation, studio photographs, and recital videos, you could easily reach the $2,000 mark. Instead of jumping the gun, put that money into a savings account. It could easily cover the tuition costs at a reputable ballet school when the child reaches age eight.

Of course, if you are only interested in the recreational and social aspects of early "ballet" training, and if money is no object —go for it! Just be really thorough in your research of the qualifications of the teacher and the content of the instruction. But if you decide to wait, and if your child does become a dancer someday, you may have saved enough for that first plane ticket to New York. *And* you will have provided her with the safe, solid foundation she will need to compete in such a fierce and demanding occupation.

BALLET FOR YOU

If you are seeking ballet training for yourself, there are a few more issues to deal with. As an adult, there are different physical limitations to consider. It is a fact that ballet is an excellent way to begin taking dance. It is the basis for all dance forms and, because of its progressive technique, can "ease" you into movement without fear of mental or physical overload. Be aware, however, of your own physical limitations. A doctor's input is essential if you have had any health problems in the past or are currently under a physician's care. It is always better to be safe than sorry.

After you have been given the green light, put your foot on the accelerator and proceed down the road to enjoyment. But remember, drive slowly and proceed with caution! You're still in driver's education, and bodies don't come equipped with seat belts and air bags.

MALE DANCERS

Up to this point I have only addressed the female would-be ballerina. What if it is your son who wants to take ballet or if you are a male wanting to take the plunge into the dance world?

Let me say this now, for the record, BEING A MALE DANCER *DOES NOT*, and I repeat, *DOES NOT* MAKE YOU A HOMOSEXUAL! Many of my male dancer friends are heterosexual, married, and have children. Yes, it is true that some male dancers do dance to the beat of a different drum; however, I don't believe for a minute that it is their love of dance that taught them the step. Unfortunately, prejudice toward men in dance, the AIDS crisis of the '80s and '90s, and people's ignorance concerning AIDS have created a major deficit in the male dance population. The fact is — anyone who is a dancer is a highly trained athlete.

Great strides have been made to recognize dancers as the great athletes that they are. I challenge any athlete or male who disputes this claim to try to perform the choreography from *A Chorus Line, Dancin'*, or *Cats* ten times a week at a performance level and come out of it alive. Male and female dancers alike now include working out daily with weights as an integral and necessary part of their training. The added strength enables them to perform the grueling feats demanded of them by directors and choreographers. It takes tremendous muscular force, endurance, and agility to dance professionally, and the male physique is well adapted to this calling. Just take a look at Mikhail Baryshnikov (and who wouldn't want to?) and try to prove me wrong. He is the ultimate in physical perfection. If I were a male in this day and age, and I had a strong desire to dance, then I would start pumping iron, head for the best dance facility I could find, and prepare for many years of joy and success. But there are a few things to watch out for on the way.

Pacing Yourself

A dance studio's biggest advertisement is its recital. The more impressive the show, the bigger the next year's enrollment. As a paying parent, it gets pretty boring to see only the girls, number after number. As a teacher, the choreographic inspirations start getting pretty lean after a dozen all-female routines. Male students in these shows give the teachers more interesting options and the audience a more varied fare. Unfortunately, boys are in the minority. In an attempt to fill the gaps at recital time, studios usually enlist the services of the fathers, brothers, and friends of their female students. Nine times out of ten, their performances are less than stellar. Thus, there is always a need for more males with training, and teachers will do almost anything to get boys in their ranks and into class. Once inside, your services will be at a premium and your ego constantly stroked. If not kept in check, this could be hazardous. To illustrate, let me tell you about my days as a youngster in ballet class.

It was supposed to be "boy/girl" time in our ballet number, but our studio was only fortunate enough to have one boy. His name was Bobby. Poor Bobby had to partner and lift every girl in our large class. Now there were some pretty big girls in my studio and, much to Bobby's dismay, they all seemed to be taking the same ballet class. Not yet having had his growth spurt and weighing in at a scant one hundred pounds, he was barely able to get most of us off the ground. Bobby wasn't a quitter, however, and with the confidence of a sumo wrestler, religiously came to class during the months prior to our recital. Every week he tested his muscle strength acting out the role of our beloved Prince. To make matters worse, and as is usually the case, Bobby was also asked to do little "bits" in other numbers, which required some of the same weightlifting skills but involved tap and jazz dancers. The night of the show rolled around and Bobby couldn't roll out of bed. Our Knight in Shining Armor had many nights in traction. Of course, after the final curtain, we all went to the hospital and fawned over him, smothering him with attention. (To this day I still believe that he would have done it all over again if he had been given the chance.) So the moral of the story is ... if you train well and don't overextend yourself, being a boy or man in a dance studio is like going to heaven! You are adored by the masses and get to watch girls run around in leotards all the time. What more could you ask for?

TEACHER QUALIFICATIONS

How do you know if the ballet teacher you are considering taking class from is really qualified? Don't be afraid to inquire about her credentials and training. It might seem like Greek to you, but you have a right to know. If the teacher cannot come up with a decent-sized list of credentials or refuses to discuss it with you because you have offended her "professionalism"—

leave. If she rattles off enough credits to pique your interest, the next step is to observe her in action and see if she does indeed know *how* to teach. Remember, all the training and stage experience in the world cannot make a good teacher. You must really watch and listen carefully to make an evaluation.

So how will you be able to ask questions or draw conclusions in order to make an intelligent decision if you feel that you are totally ignorant of dance vernacular? Whether you are a man or a woman, an adult or a child, there are some very obvious visual "tip-offs" that will help you in your quest for a ballet mentor. Again, if at all possible, you must observe the instructor teaching an actual class. That class should ideally be the one that you are considering or a class that is at or near the same level of expertise. Watching an advanced class can give you immense inspiration (or make you want to try something easier), but it will not give you a clear picture of the teacher's ability to teach beginners or of her physiology background. Advanced dancers already know their bodies and the fine art of self-correction. Thus, the instructor will probably be stressing dance combinations (steps) and performance rather than basic technique. Usually there is more than one ballet instructor at a school, and the ones who teach the lower levels do not always handle the advanced classes. Advanced classes are generally taught by the head of the studio (if ballet is her forte) or by a performing professional who can bring her special qualities and real life experience into class. Unless the studio has been in existence with the same staff for a long period of time, the advanced dancers will not give you a true representation of a specific teacher's ability. The students' initial training came from somewhere else and their base was developed under someone else's tutelage.

THE PROPER DRESS

Once allowed into the "inner sanctum," carefully observe the teaching ritual. First, take a look at the appearance of the teacher and the students. Ballet attire sets the tone and mood for a successful class, and it is the teacher's responsibility to be the role model and enforcer. If the instructor looks like she is going to be in an MTV video, or if she allows her students to dress accordingly, hightail it out of there! Self-discipline, respect for the body, and the art all go hand in hand. There are very specific reasons leotards and tights of a certain style and color were developed for the ballet class. The body, line, and alignment *are* the ballet dancer. Light pink tights originally became the "uniform" because they enabled the teacher to see the musculature of the legs through the light-colored material. They wrapped the limbs in a sleek covering that gave warmth and visibility. The leotard was developed for much the same reasons. It fit tight to the body and allowed the teacher to see the parts of the dancer's physique to ensure their proper usage. The wearing of the female's hair up and off the face in the traditional "bun" exposed the head, neck, and upper spinal areas so the teacher could monitor their use. Keeping hair out of the face also eliminated distractions.

With the growth of the exercise and dancewear industries, many studios have let their standards become lax, allowing students to wear almost anything (and sometimes almost nothing) in class. Now I am all for being progressive, and the rigid black and pink uniform of the past doesn't always work in every facility. But let's not throw all the tradition out the window. How can a new dancer discover the beauty and proper execution of a ballet movement when her body is hidden beneath layers of rock-star T-shirts and sweat pants? If you see beginning or intermediate students in a ballet class wearing loose tops, dangling jewelry, distracting exercise garb, tennis shoes (or no shoes), or tons of wild hair, it is a dead giveaway that the teacher is not professional and does not take ballet seriously.

Many studios also sell dancewear in their facilities for an added income. The more and varied dancewear you purchase and are allowed to wear in class, the higher the studio's profit. However, don't confuse the aggressive dancewear entrepreneur with the progressive dance teacher who is trying to do her clientele a real service. By buying and providing "required" classroom dancewear at lower than retail costs, or bringing supplies to her students who do not have the benefit of a nearby retail store, she is making dance more accessible to the public.

Footwear is another important issue. A ballet student must be able to feel the floor with her feet, and ballet slippers were created for this purpose. They are soft, flexible, and snug yet have a sole that gives the right amount of traction to prevent injury. The ballet slippers should have an elastic strap across the instep for safety and should not be worn with socks. The addition of a sock between the tights and shoe greatly limits the ability of the foot to meld with the floor, and if the shoe was fitted correctly to begin with, the sock would make the shoe too snug.

Pink is the preferred color for females and white for males. The light color lets the teacher see how a student uses his or her feet because worn areas indicating foot pressure can warn a teacher of a potential problem that should be corrected during the very early stages of training. In fact, a knowledgeable instructor has the uncanny ability of being able to "read" a student's ballet shoes like a navigator reads maps. There is also an aesthetic reason for the choice of pink slippers for girls and women. In combination with pink tights, they create a pleasing unbroken visual leg line, which gives an illusion of added length (a plus to any female).

For males, the desired attire consists of leotard and tights manufactured especially for the male physique. In contrast to the girls, the boys wear their leotards *under* their tights. The

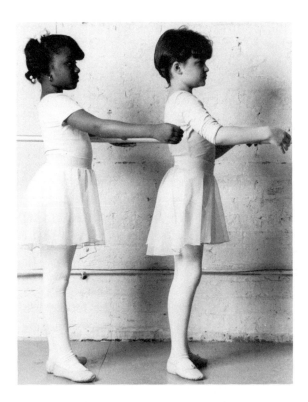

tights are made of a thicker material for obvious reasons, and a dance belt, which is similar to an athletic supporter, also helps keep the men intact and prevents injury. The leotard and tight colors are generally black and white, and you will find that your choices as a male dancewear consumer are pretty limited, especially in rural areas. However, any dance institution worth its salt should be able to mail order whatever you need if it is not readily available in your locale.

CLASS SIZE

Now take a look at class size. The number of students in a class should not be so oppressive as to limit the students' ability to use their bodies to the fullest. Too many dancers in a beginning class can result in very awkward-looking dancers who are afraid to extend themselves for fear of getting a hand in the mouth or a foot in the rear. Bad habits learned in the very early stages of training sometimes hamper a person's growth for years to come.

Private class or classes where only two or three students are in competition with each other are even less desirable than larger ones, because they can cause feelings of inadequacy or even worse, falsely inflated egos. An ideal situation would be to take a class where there is a comfortable number of students in the class, whose abilities are at both ends of the spectrum. This would give the student just the right mix of confidence, humility, and inspiration.

OBSERVING THE TEACHER

Now it's time to observe the teacher at work. Watch to see whether she pays attention to each dancer individually. Is she watching her students in the mirror or is she watching herself? Does she give corrections or make adjustments on each student or does she only address the "whole"? She should be doing both. Sometimes a blanket statement can be more effective than repeatedly singling out students of lesser competence or ability. Each person, however, is unique. There are times (at least a billion times in any dancer's training—or so it seems) when personal corrections are essential. It sometimes is embarrassing, but there is really no other way to teach.

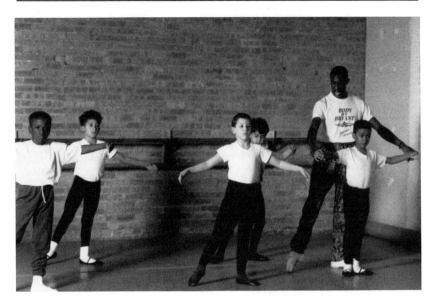

Terminology

The specific corrections that you should be looking for might need a little explanation. They concern *alignment* and *turn-out*. Let me give you a crash cour se on both. Aside from being something that you have adjusted on your car, good alignment is the foundation for every good dancer, and it can be understood quite easily. Think of your car again. If it is out of alignment, the whole thing is crooked. It puts stress on the wrong parts and does not allow the car to function properly. The same is true in dance. A dancer's body has three main heavy parts—the head, torso, and pelvis. If these three sections are not "aligned" when a dancer moves, there will be injury and imbalance.

The teacher should constantly be watching for heads that are bent down (usually watching the feet), swayed backs or hunched shoulders, and pelvises that are either pushing out to the rear or tucking under to the front. All three "sections" should be lined up, one on top of the other, like three spools of thread. The center of these spools should be perfectly aligned so that a pencil could be inserted down the middle. When a dancer achieves this positioning on her own, she has found her "center." Obviously, in the initial stages of dance, this process must be taught, and it is vital that the teacher gives each student the tools to align his or her own vehicle. If the body is kept in alignment, the dancer will function like a finely tuned automobile and stay out of the repair shop.

"Turn-out" of the feet in ballet class is the big issue. It is not accomplished, and I cannot stress this enough, by a student simply standing with her feet pointing outwards in the five basic foot positions. True and lasting turn-out comes from the hip sockets (ouch!). Beginning the movement in this area allows the knees and feet to follow naturally (if you consider it natural) without injury. This point has to be stressed and the execution policed during a ballet class, or the students may end up ruining their knees and backs. The actual rotation of the hip sockets to achieve proper turn-out should not be taught or begun before the age of eight or so, when a child's bones and muscles are ready to handle this adjustment. Good turn-out takes a very long time to achieve, and a qualified teacher will regulate her students' attempts to reach this goal.

While you are watching for turn-out also keep an eye out for the overdevelopment of calves and thighs. If a large percentage of the legs look as if they belong on "Big Time Wrestling," it could be an indication that there has been some bad training along the way. You should be able to see an advanced dancer's musculature when she is dancing, not when she is standing at rest. A dancer's body is built of strength *and* stretch. Think about the enviable figures of most professional dancers, and you will realize that there is no room for bulky muscles in such a visual art form.

The only way to determine if the teacher in question was the muscle builder is to ask if the "bulky" students have had training elsewhere. If the instructor boasts of being their only teacher and that they are his or her "prize" students, be very careful. They could have brought their large limbs with them or could participate in other activities that might be increasing their muscular volume (excessive use of weights, bad running or jogging techniques, etc.), or the teacher could be deficient in the knowledge of physiology. Exercise caution! Should you be unable to draw a conclusion and choose to enroll in that teacher's class, monitor your own body's progress carefully. If you start resembling Rambo (especially if you are female), look for the nearest exit.

OTHER DETERMINING FACTORS

There may be a couple of other things to look for, which, if present in a young beginner's class, might help "tip the scales." The first would be the presence of "assistants" or "demonstrators." It is almost impossible for an instructor in a beginner class (especially one with a lot of students) to be able to catch and correct all the mistakes going on at any particular moment. Assistants can either free up the teacher by doing the movements during the exercises (so the students can follow them), which lets the teacher walk around and fix mistakes, or they can adjust the students in conjunction with the primary instructor. The end result is that the students' errors are not overlooked. My own daughter's ballet teacher uses two such assistants, and I find it really gratifying to see my daughter constantly given the personal attention. I really believe that it benefits all concerned.

The other plus to look for is the presence of live musical accompaniment. If there is a piano in class, it not only adds a richness to the experience, but it also keeps the class moving because the teacher doesn't have to constantly stop and find music. You will be getting more instruction for your money.

WRAP-UP

Finding the right ballet class is not really as difficult a task as it seems. Before you decide to hang your "slippers" from your car mirror and take up basket weaving instead, let me make it really simple. When trying to choose the right ballet class, ask yourself these few questions:

❑ Is the ballet class right for the age, ability, and physical limitations of the student?
❑ Does the teacher have solid credentials?
❑ Do the teacher and students dress properly for class?
❑ Is the class the desirable size?
❑ Is attention paid to each student individually?
❑ Does the teacher stress alignment and proper turn-out?
    If the answer to all these questions is YES, then put on your ballet slippers and leap into dance school. You will have a great flight!

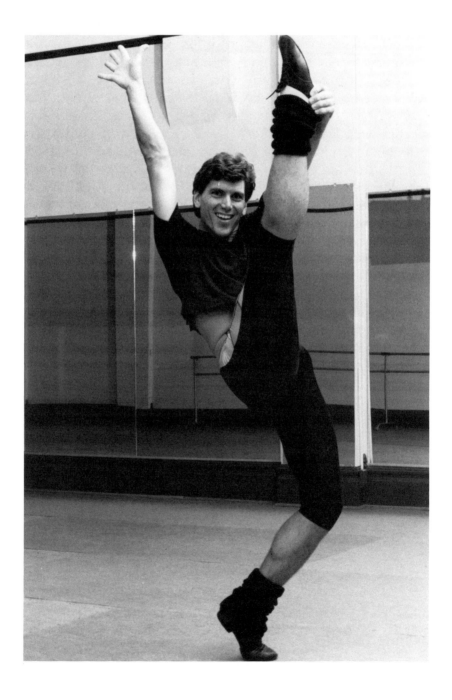

9
All That Jazz

I love the sense of movement, the sense of freedom ... If you execute a
dance step, there is a sense of flying."
Bob Fosse

J azz dance or modern jazz (as it is sometimes called) is almost impossible to describe. It encompasses many different dance forms and cultures and can consist of any combination of African dance, modern dance, rock, musical theater, current dance styles, and ballet. It is sometimes set to the soul-searching pulses of a conga drum, the electrifying music that excites the younger generation, old standards, hot jazz, or Broadway show tunes. But no matter where the moves come from or what music or accompaniment they are choreographed to, one thing is for sure—jazz dance has a rhythm, a beat, a sexuality, and a flow that no other dance form can hold a candle to! Every part of the body gets to move, sometimes in isolation or all at the same time. Good jazz is fun, constantly changing, and mentally and physically challenging. I love it!

WHEN TO START

The only real problems lie in when and where to start. Age is an important consideration. Since the styles of jazz vary so greatly, certain types require a more "adult" body. I feel that, as in ballet, age eight is the youngest age at which to start taking lessons. Before this age, the body is usually not mature enough to handle the complex moves and concepts of this fast-paced dance form. I also believe, as do most of my peers, that ballet should be taken at the same time or introduced soon thereafter. The combination of the two is necessary if a person wants to progress to the upper levels and beyond, and many studios wisely require students above a beginner level to take companion ballet instruction in order to gain admittance into higher level classes. Be sure to check with each administrator as to the studio's policies. Additional classes are not free, and if money is a serious consideration, you will want to know what you're getting into right at the start.

You are never too old for jazz as long as you know your own physical limitations and are assured that the teacher is competent and qualified. If you are the least bit concerned about your ability to survive, it would be wise to check with your doctor before beginning any activity that involves major movement. One thing is for sure—jazz certainly does.

WHAT TYPE OF JAZZ?

Now that you are ready to begin, how do you decide which type of jazz you want to explore and how do you find a knowledgeable "guide?" Jazz dance varies drastically from teacher to teacher, class to class, studio to studio, and state to state, so choosing your "point of departure" involves some visual detective work. You are going to have to observe more than one school or studio in order to better acquaint yourself with the types of styles that are available in your area. However, to get a feel for each studio, you do not have to attend a lot of individual classes. It is more beneficial, less time consuming, and a heck of a lot more fun to attend local dance recitals, performances, and concerts. Go for the entertainment value. Sit back and relax. You will know when you have come across a jazz style that's right because your hips will start swaying and your fingers will start snapping. If you are not inspired, look further until you really get the desire to join in. Each person will react differently to the same style, and what's right for some might be all wrong for you, so let your soul tell you what *you* want to learn. Jazz dance comes from within and should feel good. To quote one of my favorite songs: "It don't mean a thing if it ain't got that swing."

So now you have found an intriguing style, and you're just itching to feel the beat. How can you tell if the teacher knows his stuff and is the right one for you? This is where *individual* teacher and class observation is important. Go to the school or studio and watch the prospective instructors in action. If this is not possible because classes are not in session yet or the teacher is new, go ahead and sign up and do your evaluation during the first few classes. Just be sure that you can withdraw without losing any money. When in the class, you will have to put all the visual stimuli aside and look at the class *content* to make an appraisal. No matter what the style, jazz class can basically be divided into two parts—warmup and combinations.

WARMUP

Let's talk about warmup first. Each instructor will take his own personal knowledge and background and adapt them to his particular jazz style. Thus, each teacher's warmup varies considerably from that of other teachers. A warmup *must* be part of the class, however, or the class is dangerous and the teacher negligent. Jazz places special demands on the body, and no amount of normal activity can prepare someone to dance. Think of your body as your car again, on a cold winter's day. It takes a lot of idling before it can run efficiently. The mechanics of the body are similar, in that the parts must be sufficiently warmed up and the joints lubricated before you try to put them through their paces. This pre-movement stretch should be comprehensive and lengthy, and approximately one-third to one-half of the class should be devoted to these moves. Warmup is the time when a person not only prepares muscles for the vigorous and demanding combinations that will follow, but where basic technique and terminology are also drilled and mastered. It gets the mind into "dance mode" and gets rid of tension, so a student can leave the real world and its problems outside of the dance class where they belong.

While watching different classes, you will see that stretching can be done in many different ways—at the barre, standing, sitting, lying on the floor, in front of the mirror, or all of the above. No matter how it is done, the warmup should begin slowly with controlled movements that allow the body to ease into motion safely. Also watch for teacher direction. During a beginning or intermediate student level warmup, the teacher should explain the stretches as they are executed and should be correcting and *gently* adjusting each student when necessary to avoid injury. Major force should never be applied. Occasionally, you will see warmups done as a continual routine. These types of warmups are very effective but should only be used in more advanced class situations where the students have acquired the knowledge to correct themselves. There is no time in a choreographed warmup routine to stop and make the corrections that are so very necessary in the formative classes, so if the warmup in a *beginner* student class looks like a recital piece, be very cautious.

DANCEWEAR

While we are on the subject of corrections, let's talk about dancewear. A teacher can't correct what he can't see, so beware of the teacher who allows beginning and intermediate students into class wearing baggy clothes or streetwear. The instructor who permits students to take class without proper dancewear is not only doing a great disservice to his pupils but to dance in general. Teaching professionalism and respect for the art is as important as teaching the craft, so if an instructor is lax in the dancewear area or validates inappropriate behavior by dressing improperly for class himself, you should look elsewhere. Loose-fitting trendy dance looks (i.e., big T-shirts, sweat shirts, sweat pants, etc.) are also not appropriate in novice classes. Again, remember, if it can't be seen, it can't be corrected.

It has become harder and harder in recent years to keep fashion's influence out of the lower level classes because jazz, by its very nature, inspires wild clothing. All you have to do is walk into a professional class to know this to be true. In fact, some of the outfits that the pros wear have to be seen to be believed. There will be plenty of time, however, to draw attention to yourself after you have mastered the art and really have something to show off. Until then, form-fitting dancewear (though it may be more boring) is the right choice.

FOOTWEAR

The jazz oxford was created specifically for jazz class and is worn by both males and females. It looks like a very soft tennis shoe, but it is extremely flexible, and the sole is designed to accommodate a variety of movements. The lace-up style is more stable than the strap type (which resembles a soft Mary Jane) because it is more form-fitting. The shoe is made of either canvas or leather but the choice of material is more a matter of esthetic preference than of function. The bottom can be either suede or rubber to accommodate different floor surfaces.

Some studios allow ballet slippers in jazz class but I do not recommend them. I feel that they have a tendency to slip off; they do not wear well under the rigors of jazz; and they don't give an impressionable, inexperienced dancer the right jazz "feel." I am also not at all fond of sneakers because of their inflexibility, which does not allow for the full use of the foot and the development of the "pointe." The thick rubber bottom also sticks to most floor surfaces and can easily give a student a nasty ankle or knee injury.

One shoe to definitely watch out for is the heeled character shoe. This shoe looks like a heeled tap shoe with a strap across the instep and has *no* place in beginner classes. These are for advanced students or pros who are required to wear these types of footwear in performance. They can be very dangerous on the feet of the inexperienced, and no reputable teacher would allow them at the lower levels.

Some teachers have the students warm up barefoot. This is an accepted practice and makes it easier for a student to work his feet and arches and lets the toes "feel" the floor, which promotes proper weight placement. It also lets the instructor watch the feet more carefully to discourage any bad habits from forming. Once the warmup is complete, however, the students should put on shoes to finish the rest of the class safely.

No matter what is worn on the feet during the warmup, be sure that there is a warmup and that the students are dressed appropriately to get the most out of their class and to allow the teacher to correct them individually.

TEACHING TECHNIQUES

Before we get to the actual dancing, there is another teaching technique that you may encounter, which might need some clarification. Many jazz instructors follow the warmup with traveling moves or combinations in which the students dance from one side of the room to the other or from corner to corner (to cover more distance). This helps the students get their brains and bodies "into gear" before having to tackle and retain more complex combinations or routines. It also serves as a refresher course in basic jazz steps and techniques and, since the moves are usually executed individually or "two at a time," it gives the teacher a chance to evaluate and work with each student independently. I employ this technique when I teach. I feel that it can be very beneficial, not only in strengthening the basics, but also in building up the confidence of the novice dancer by putting him "on the line" and making him dance solo without the safety net of anonymity provided by dancing with his classmates.

COMBINATIONS

Now comes the second half of the class and the fun part—the REAL dancing. It can either be in the form of isolated combinations (series of steps that are not part of an actual performance piece) or steps that are part of an ongoing routine the students are expected to retain for a recital, show, or performance. It is my belief that students should be exposed to both. Too many lower level studios concentrate solely on pieces for their recitals, which are one of their main sources of income. Constant drilling on this material makes for a precision performance, but it can be monotonous and make class unchallenging and mundane. Concentrating only on performance routines can also limit a student's progression into higher levels of expertise, because it does not give a firm technical foundation or equip students with the fast comprehensive skills that they will need later on down the line for auditions and professional theater. A school that knows the benefits of a good base, constant stimuli, and challenge and combines them with *occasional* performance will give a well-rounded dance education. One that is concerned only with recital routines and studio revenue makes its students pay dearly, in the end, for all those sequins. There will be plenty of time to strut your stuff. Be patient. Rome wasn't built in a day but it was built on a strong foundation!

The content of the combinations or routines is not as important as the teacher's ability to teach them and to structure them to the right level of students. Focus on the instructor's methods. While teaching a step, he should dissect each movement, count out each step, and explain it over and over again until the majority of the class has gotten the hang of it. Remember, we are talking about beginners here. It takes tons of patience and a lot of repetition. Not everyone is going to pick up the steps with the same speed, so it is necessary to break down the combinations repeatedly until most of the students can perform them adequately. If after an entire class, however, the majority of the students are *really* struggling, and they look more confused, frustrated, and depressed than exhilarated, it could be an indicator that the teacher does not know the "pulse" of the class and is not adept at teaching beginners.

Don't get me wrong. The steps should be a challenge, but by the end of a session most of the students should have risen to the occasion and should be experiencing a feeling of accomplishment. That's really important, especially in novice classes where self-esteem is at an all-time low. A good teacher will know his students' levels and backgrounds and will choreograph accordingly. He will be supportive and give encouragement, and any criticism or corrections will be given constructively, keeping his students' lack of experience in mind. After all, dance class is supposed to be fun and rewarding, not ego-shattering. If the students look miserable after class, it's the teacher's doing. Look for another class—one that you will look forward to attending week after week.

WRAP-UP

❏ Find the style of jazz that feels good to you.
❏ Evaluate the instructor and class.
❏ Look for a professional atmosphere with appropriate dress.
❏ There should be a safe, progressive, comprehensive warm-up followed by a rewarding session of dance.

If you find all these things, then join in the fun. You will get a great workout for your brain and body, eliminate stress, and get to know yourself better than you could ever have imagined. As your inhibitions melt away and the music takes over your soul, a newly confident person will emerge. But I must warn you—once bitten by the jazz bug there is no turning back! Who would want to?

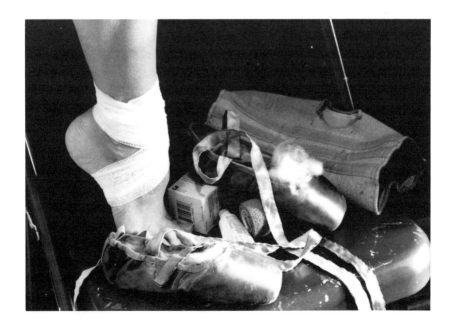

10
What's the Pointe?

It is a fine thing to build your castles in the air as long as your
foundations are on the ground.
Henry David Thoreau

You might wonder why I made an entire separate chapter on pointe and why I did not include it in the section on ballet. It's because toe dancing is in a category all by itself. It is not an amateur sport!

Since this guide is basically for beginners, there should really be no need to mention pointe at all except that, as a teacher, I have always wanted to air my opinions publicly and, as parents or prospective students, you must be educated about the dangers of premature pointe work. Some dance instructors are going to be really ticked off with me for this, but I am going to stick my neck out and say what I firmly believe. *No one should go on pointe unless they have serious aspirations and a burning desire to become a professional dancer.* If you are passionate about such a career, have studied seriously for many, many years, take ballet class *at least* three times a week, have been given the go-ahead by a qualified teacher, and are studying at a school that specializes in ballet and whose teachers know their stuff, *then* learning to dance on toe is necessary to realize your dreams. If not— don't do it!

When most girls get enamored with ballet they are viewing it through rose-colored glasses. In the back of their minds lurk glittering fantasies of dancing on pointe wearing fluffy tutus and rhinestone tiaras to the spellbinding strains of Swan Lake. What they fail to realize, however, is that it takes an incredible amount of training, strength, and dedication even to begin dancing on toe. Many students and their parents believe that as soon as they hit puberty it is their *right* to don pointe shoes. It is not a right. It is a privilege that should not be granted to the amateur dancer.

MEDICAL REASONS FOR DELAYING POINTE WORK

Dr. Richard H. Dominguez, Orthopedic Surgeon and author of *The Complete Book of Sports Medicine*, believes that "pointe work shouldn't begin until a girl is fully grown, which is usually two years after the start of her period." He told me that "some teachers are even becoming increasingly cautious and are requiring signed 'permission notes' from an orthopedic surgeon verifying that the prospective toe student has acquired sufficient hip socket turn-out before allowing them to participate in pointe work." Bully for them! Dr. Dominguez also observed that a lot of parents and dancers are not realistic about their bodies and dance goals. "A female has to have 'the perfect body' for ballet and one who is too leggy, overweight, short, or top or bottom heavy is just not suited for a career on pointe and would be better off trying a different dance form." Ballet and pointe do not have to follow each other. Ballet, in and of itself, is the basis for all dance and should be mastered to give a dancer a solid foundation.

For some stupid reason, many, many parents think that dancing on pointe elevates (no pun intended) their daughter in the eyes of other students, neighbors, and relatives and that it has to be the end result of a couple of years of recreational ballet classes. In turn, they put constant pressure on teachers to advance their children prematurely. I know from experience that one of the things that frustrates and angers teachers most is pushy parents who believe that *they* know what's right for their child's dance "career" and insist that little Susie be allowed to dance in toe shoes even when she is not old enough or isn't prepared. Some even threaten to withdraw their child from the studio if their demands are not met. What is really tragic, however, is that there are many money hungry, irresponsible dance instructors out there who cave in to the whim of these starstruck parents, or who are just not knowledgeable enough in their craft, and put children through years of unnecessary pain and frustration just to earn a buck. These teachers let students who take only one student level ballet class a week wobble blissfully around wrecking their ankles, feet, knees, backs, or internal organs as they grin, hand out hollow accolades, and smile all the way to the bank! If it sounds like I'm being a little harsh, I am!

INSTRUCTOR QUALIFICATIONS

Pointe instruction should be given by only the most highly qualified ballet instructors. If a neighborhood dance studio's curriculum is made up of mainly tap and jazz classes, then there probably aren't enough high level ballet classes being offered

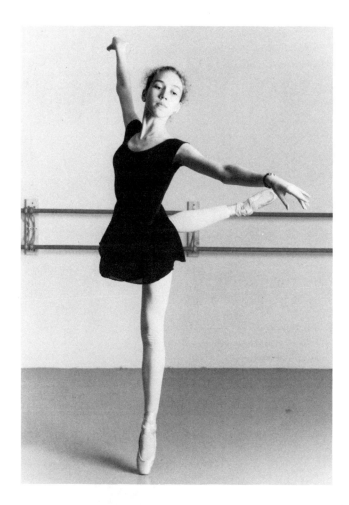

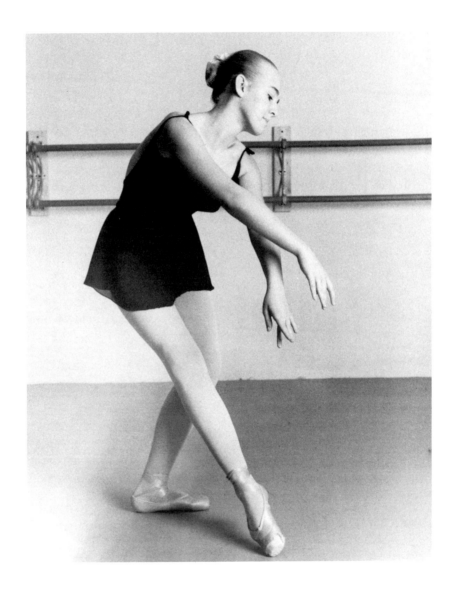

each week to supply a serious ballet student with the necessary amount of continual training required (at least three high level classes per week) to keep the student technically strong enough to handle the rigors of pointe. Ballet is probably not the forte of the teachers at this type of facility either, so you would be wise to seek toe and ballet instruction elsewhere.

My feeling has always been that when you want something done right, you should go to an expert or a specialist in the field. If ballet is your "thing," then you should be in a ballet school. Round out your career if you like by taking other types of classes, but take your ballet and pointe classes at a reputable school that specializes in ballet and that has the concentrated courses and performing outlets that you will need. There is no law that says you cannot take from two studios at the same time, and no one teacher or studio can give you all that you need to be a well-rounded dancer. You need to study many different places and under the trained eye of numerous instructors with varied backgrounds to become competent in your chosen field. Take off the rose-colored glasses and believe me, you will get a clearer picture of reality.

WRAP-UP

If you or your child are only dancing for fun, recreation, and the social benefits of dance rather than to gain the skills needed for a possible ballet career, don't push yourself or your daughter onto pointe. It is unnecessary, potentially dangerous, and expensive. A lot of studio and dancewear store revenue will be lost when parents finally wake up and smell the coffee, but I for one can't wait for the day when pointe is recognized as the specialty that it is. It should be taught selectively and only by those who have the training and qualifications to teach it correctly.

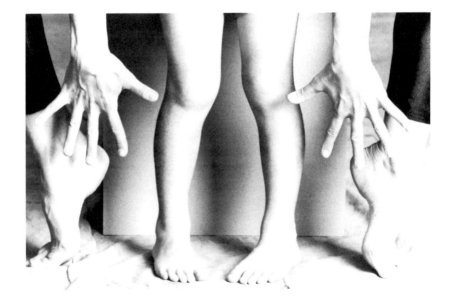

11
Modern Dance

*Dance is the only art in which we ourselves are
the stuff of which it is made.*
Ted Shawn

Do you long to dance barefoot through life? Are you fascinated by motion and movement? Does your soul soar by nature and do your emotions run rampant and your feelings flow freely? If so, then modern dance could be for you.

Modern dance is "organic"—truly an expression of all movement. Unlike ballet, there are few rules and those that exist are meant to be broken. Unlike jazz, it is an internal quest rather than an external celebration. It is based on personal communication with oneself and others and can run the gamut from creative movement classes for children to almost mystical, soul-searching, interpretive courses for adults. If you or your child want to move for movement's sake and want to be an integral part of the creative process, then modern dance is just the ticket.

Classes can be enjoyed by either sex, can be begun at any age, and, as long as there is an adequate warmup, you will find the moves are so natural that there is little chance of injury. It is because of its natural progression that modern dance and creative movement classes are the perfect way to introduce young children to movement. It makes so much more sense to let them explore dance by using their inner creativity and openness than to put them in rigidly structured ballet classes prematurely. Rules go against their very nature, and the nature of modern dance is NO RULES. Little children love to move, and they do it with such gusto and total abandon. There is plenty of time to harness them and direct their energies *after* the love of movement has developed strong roots. Creative movement can give them these roots and, what is even more important, it is fun!

BEGINNING MOVEMENT CLASSES

By using rhythmic games, "mirroring," basic movements, and stretches, young students learn about their own bodies and how they move through space. Levels, tempos, direction, and shapes are explored both alone and in relation to other members of the group, and this exploration is done naturally with very little structure. Creative movement, if taught properly, can be a rewarding experience for a young child. Introducing dance through this medium makes the other forms of dance that follow more enjoyable and productive because the kids are not "burnt out" by premature overexposure to structure and technique by the ripe old age of eight.

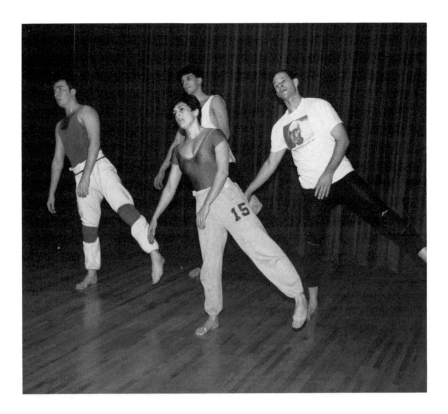

MODERN DANCE IS FOR EVERYONE

Many, many adults have also discovered that they have a real love for movement by starting their dance training in modern classes. It "grounds" you and gives you inner vision while teaching you how to communicate thought, feelings, and ideas through motion.

Older students will go on the same exploration as their young creative movement counterparts, adding their maturity and vast array of personal experiences to take the understanding of the human body to new heights. You will delve into the four basic elements of dance—body, force, space, and time— while learning modern dance technique and patterns giving you a whole new insight into movement. Modern dance is for all people no matter what background, age, or body type.

Men seem to enjoy this form of movement as much as women do, and, even though the females still outnumber them, males are willingly signing up for modern classes. For some reason, a man's masculinity doesn't seem as threatened in modern dance. This could be because the majority of courses are offered at colleges and universities where there is less stigma than at isolated private dance facilities. Modern dance is "just another course" to many academic students, and they sign up with the intention of fulfilling a physical education requirement, never dreaming that they might get hooked along the way. Upon course completion, however, many find that they wish to continue or want to explore other types of dance. In fact, some of the world's best male dancers started out exactly that way.

WHERE TO FIND CLASSES

Most colleges offer modern dance classes. They can be taken for credit or fun, and these facilities usually have good instructors, a wide variety of class levels for both children and adults, and they may even offer performing opportunities. Some dance studios have also added modern dance to their curriculum, and there are many top-notch schools that specialize exclusively in this form of dance. When you find a facility, try to observe the prospective teacher and class before signing up to determine whether they are the right ones for you.

OBSERVING CLASSES

Modern classes should begin with a comprehensive warmup. Warmups usually begin on the floor or at the barre and should be progressive in their movements, beginning slowly with controlled motions, and working up to larger and faster ones. This type of preparation is necessary to avoid injuring cold muscles. It also gets the students mentally ready to dance.

The moves will generally be accompanied by the beat of a drum or claves (a pair of wooden sticks that are hit together to produce a beat) or, if you are lucky, by a pianist or live musicians. Sometimes records, tapes, or compact discs are used, depending on the desired feel or desired results. It is completely the preference of the teacher as to which type of accompaniment is used. Just be sure that there is some form of rhythmic beat or music being used in the class (especially in beginner situations) since learning rhythm is one of the main objectives.

Watch for the teacher to make individual corrections concerning body and weight placement and correct step execution. No one is going to do it correctly all the time, so there should be a lot of adjusting and verbal instruction going on. These corrections should be constructive in nature and should be balanced out by frequent words of encouragement and praise.

CLASS STRUCTURE AND MOVEMENT

Look for an actual "structure" to the class content. By this I mean to be wary of beginner classes that look like all improvisation— the ones where people run around pretending to be trees and flowers for an hour. Modern dance, though freer than other dance styles, does have a definite technique that must be presented and mastered in order to understand the body and how it moves. If the class seems to make no sense, it probably won't make sense for you to take it. Look elsewhere.

What should the actual movements look like? As you locate courses, you will find that, like jazz, there are many different styles of modern from which to choose. Each instructor's technique will vary based on the teachings of one or more famous modern dance "gurus" (Martha Graham, Doris Humphrey, Merce Cunningham, Mary Wigman, etc.) to which she adds her own personal knowledge and experience to make it unique.

Each will have a "life of its own," depending not only on the instructor, but on the participating students and their backgrounds and the individuality that each will bring to the class. All the styles are legitimate. It is not a matter of *what* they should look like as much as what they should *feel* like to you. You may have to try a few on for size before you find the perfect fit; however, most modern dance classes aren't oppressively expensive so it won't send you to the poorhouse.

SUPPLIES

Regular form-fitting dancewear is required for class, though footless or "stirrup" tights (tights that have no feet but are held down under the arch with a sling) are generally substituted for the usual leg attire. Having the feet exposed helps the dancers work more closely with the floor, and many students simply cut off the bottom part of a pair of old tights to achieve the desired results. Men's tights are thicker and can be worn alone or under tight jazz pants or a unitard. The uniform is then topped off with a T-shirt. A dance belt (a specially designed supporter) should also be worn by both men and boys to prevent injury.

Shoes are sometimes used, and a specific modern sandal was created that protects the ball of the foot while exposing the toes and heel. It's always a good idea to wait until you get into class before you purchase shoes because some teachers are purists and prefer that you dance without them.

WRAP-UP

Modern dance is for everyone—from preschoolers on up. Look for classes at the local university or at a private dance studio. Observe classes for progressive, comprehensive warmups, musical accompaniment to develop knowledge of rhythm, and constructive individual corrections. Classes should have a definite structure.

If you take modern dance one thing is for sure—you'll bare more than your feet, you will bare your soul. It will be a revelation and an experience you will never regret!

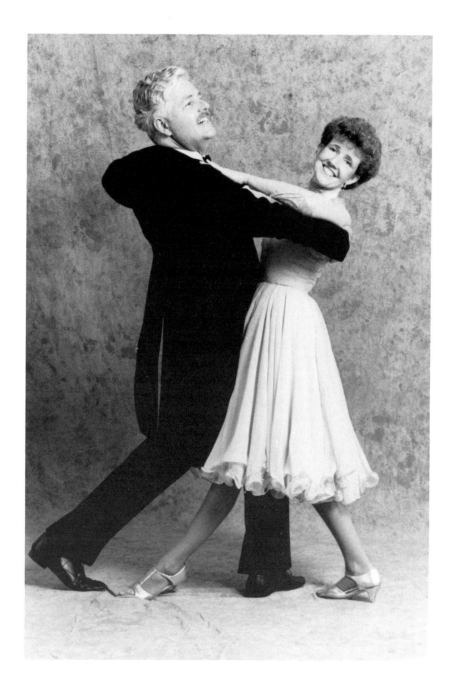

12
Ballroom

I could have danced, danced, danced all night.
My Fair Lady

It has always been a fantasy of mine to be Ginger Rogers. What girl wouldn't want to be swept around the floor dancing cheek to cheek with the likes of Fred Astaire? For that matter, what man wouldn't want to possess the suave, debonair moves of Fred himself? I really believe that romance would come back into fashion if everyone could ballroom dance. Imagine the possibilities—husbands and wives actually going out on the town and dancing the night away. There would be no more bowling dates or couch potatoes. Men would gladly dress up (the impossible dream), and women would wear flowing gowns that flattered their figures instead of jeans and sweat shirts.

I must admit that I did not acquire this infatuation with ballroom dancing until college. When I was first introduced to it at the ripe old age of nine or so, I was less than thrilled. Going to ballroom class meant wearing itchy party dresses, tight white gloves, and being "the boy." One thing is certain, there are never enough boys in ballroom class and if you're unfortunate enough to be tall as a child, you may suffer the weekly indignity of "leading" and learning the steps backwards (two habits that can haunt you for the rest of your life). At nine I was almost my full height of 5'7" (four feet of which was legs), and I weighed in at about eighty pounds. For what seemed like hours, I would maneuver my female partner around the floor trying not to look totally ridiculous. It really wasn't a very enjoyable experience.

When I took ballroom again in college, however, my entire attitude did a "one-eighty." Ballroom was a segment of my Dance

Dance History course, which began with Medieval dance and ended with the current social dance styles. My instructor was not a qualified ballroom teacher, so she wisely enlisted the aid of a professional in the field. I don't remember what his name was, but suffice it to say, he was a Latin hunk! Not only did he resemble a lithe young Ricardo Montalban, but he moved with the grace of a panther. I had the honor (much to the dismay of my other classmates) of being his partner. To this day I have no idea why I was lucky enough to be chosen, but I am sure glad I was. Never before had I experienced the feeling of being in someone's complete control. He was so expert at leading that as long as I didn't forget the footwork, we moved as one smooth entity. It was like dying and going to heaven! The experience was so memorable that I have been trying for many years to talk my husband into taking ballroom classes with me. (I figure every marriage can use all the sparks it can get.) I am convinced that if you master ballroom techniques, your life will take on a whole new meaning, and if you are lucky enough to have a comparable partner, you are going to have a great time.

THE SCOPE OF BALLROOM DANCE

In today's dance world, the term "ballroom dancing" can mean many different things. Classes can cover the old basics (i.e., waltz, cha-cha, fox trot, polka, swing, etc.), the current dance crazes, Latin styles, and even western dance. You may find that you will need to study with more than one instructor to acquire a wide range of skills. Many neighborhood studios and community centers offer ballroom classes, and there are also the better known "franchised" studios and national chains that specialize in this type of dance.

Almost all the classes will be in the evenings or on weekends, so that they are convenient for adults. Ballroom classes are generally geared toward a more mature clientele and because of its very nature, should not be introduced until a child is in his or her teens. The problem is that most normal preteens lack the self-confidence to relate comfortably in a boy/girl situation, because everybody still has "cooties." There is no real reason to rush this instruction, unless, of course, the child's social status requires these skills. Come on, what normal ten year old needs to learn to cha-cha? Let him play softball instead. Once a person is a young adult, however, ballroom dancing can give him added confidence and valuable social skills, and can increase his own physical awareness.

On the other side of the coin, ballroom dancing is a wonderful way for seniors to socialize, get exercise, and meet new friends. There are many, many clubs and organizations that older citizens can join that not only give instruction but also plan dancing activities. It is never too late to learn. In fact, many retirees now list ballroom dancing as one of their primary social outlets.

The Problem of Con Artists

I must, however, put a damper on things and warn you about con artists. Unfortunately, there are unscrupulous business people out there who prey on naive clientele. Unsuspecting lonely single people are their targets, and many of these victims are female and senior citizens. Do not sign contracts, and whenever possible, take class as part of a group instead of privately. It is a lot more fun to take instruction with a bunch of people; it helps in overcoming shyness; and it could keep you out of a compromising situation. I am not implying for a moment that *all* ballroom studios have questionable practices. Even though the majority are reputable and offer high quality instruction, some rip-off schools do exist. If you are the least bit suspicious or feel uncomfortable, check with the local Better Business Bureau to see if anyone has lodged a complaint. They should be able to give you a clearer insight into a company's track record, and if that doesn't work, try your city Chamber of Commerce.

MEN ON THE DANCE FLOOR

If you are male and are considering ballroom dance, put your inhibitions aside and go for it! The women in your life will thank you tenfold. Imagine how it will feel to be constantly in demand at social functions and the envy of all your bench-warmer friends. I guarantee that your self-confidence will increase with every dip. In fact, I am planning on enrolling my own son, Matt, as soon as he's ready, and I can't wait to see the look of gratitude on his bride's face. He will never do a bad variation of the twist at his wedding!

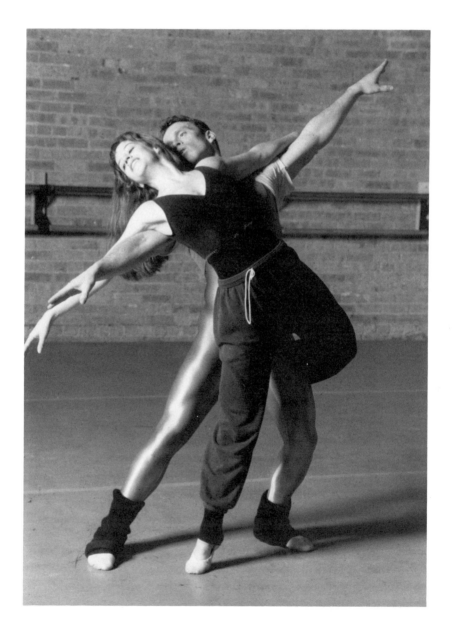

studios offer special "package" rates (i.e., eight weeks for $40) or group or senior discounts. Just be sure not to sign up for additional instruction as a prerequisite to getting these reduced rates. It is important to know what you're getting into.

APPROPRIATE DRESS

There are no specific dancewear requirements, though both men and women should wear clothes that have plenty of room for movement. Regular dance practice clothes are acceptable, especially if the class will be more advanced and contain athletic-type spins and lifts, but the traditional "out on the town" attire would probably be more comfortable for the beginner student or senior who is interested in the tamer forms of social dancing. Most instructors prefer that female students wear one-piece dresses as opposed to skirts with tops, which may have a tendency to creep up and bare the middle. Full skirts are best to allow for a full range of movement, and dance trunks (a thick-knit dance brief) should be worn underneath to avoid embarrassment during turns, spins, and dips. Street shoes or dance shoes with a medium heel are best, and they should have an instep or ankle strap for security and a sole that won't stick to the surface of the studio floor.

Men should wear comfortable slacks and shirts, and a jacket is optional unless required by the studio. Shoes should be of a dressier type, preferably with ties for security and, like the women's, have a sole that is appropriate for the floor of the studio. Each individual teacher will have his or her own preferences, so it is always wise to inquire at registration as to what clothing is acceptable.

WRAP-UP

Once you have mastered the steps, it won't really matter what you wear. You will feel confident to grab a partner and head for the dance floor. On second thought, maybe you could have a special shirt made for those nights out on the town. It could have big bold letters on it that say ... Fred and Ginger, EAT YOUR HEARTS OUT!

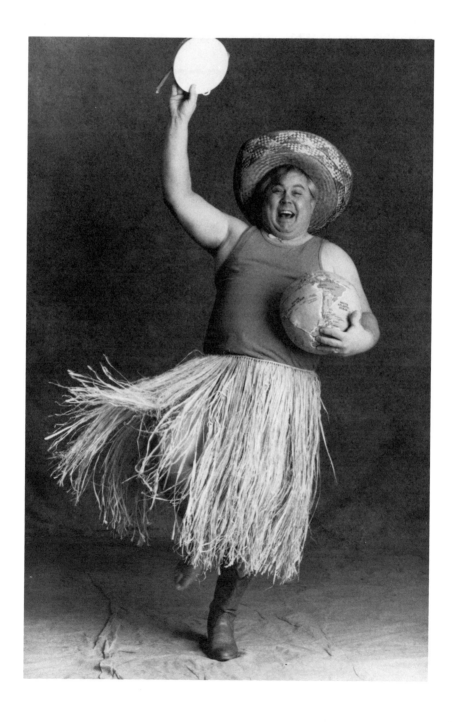

13
Folk and Ethnic

The truest expression of a people is in its dances and its music.
Agnes DeMille

Like most American "mutts," my own roots are a tangled mix of many different nationalities. When asked my heritage, however, I have a shameful tendency to "go for the gold" and only lay claim to the more impressive lineage or notorious relatives from the more glamorous places. It's much more fun talking about my ancestor who was a martyr priest from Alsace-Lorraine and who was beheaded in Tonkin than it is telling of the everyday exploits of my great, great uncle, the dentist.

The truth of the matter (and one that most people often forget) is that all people, no matter what their occupation, have a beautiful, rich heritage. Each person plays an integral part in shaping a society, and each society has a wealth of customs and traditions. Dance is one of the strongest. Delving into ethnic movement can give you a whole new insight into your past, can introduce you to a new culture, and will undoubtedly enrich your life. My uncle's job may not have been thrilling, but his Dutch blood flowing through my veins fills me with pride and creates a lasting bond between myself and the hard-working people who wore wooden shoes and linen caps. To learn and master their dance would be the ultimate compliment to my ancestors, and someday I hope to be able to indulge myself. When I do, it is comforting to know that I won't have to go overseas for instruction. I will be able to learn their dance right here. You too can travel the world without leaving home, by taking classes in ethnic or folk dance. Its masters are everywhere. You just need to know where to find them.

LOCATING TEACHERS

I cannot begin to talk about all ethnic dance forms. They are as numerous and varied as the people themselves. What I can do, however, is give you a general idea of where to start. You will find that deciding what type of dance to study is a lot easier than finding a class or an instructor. The obvious place to begin is the neighborhood dance school. A few phone calls will tell you if what you are looking for is readily available. If not, you will have to be a little more creative with your approach.

Classes in the more popular types of ethnic and folk dance (i.e., Hawaiian, Tahitian, Spanish, Irish, Greek, Middle Eastern, and Asian) will be easier to locate. Most metropolitan areas have communities with heavy concentrations of ethnic groups, and each of these "little cities" has recreational facilities, annual celebrations, and promotional councils. If, for instance, you have a yearning to learn Oriental dance, a visit to Chinatown would be in order. If you are dying to learn the *misirlou*, take a trek to Greektown. Most cultural areas have ethnic festivals that feature traditional dancers and, with some polite inquiries, could easily provide you with the names and numbers of dance instructors.

The St. Patrick's Day Parade would be a great way to tap into the network of Irish dance teachers, and "Little Italy" is sure to have many festivals where you could locate an expert on the tarantella. The Tourist Information Center of each city or state can help you with the dates and locations of their annual ethnic celebrations, and they may also be able to give you the names of the coordinator of each event. These organizers will know where the entertainment for each festival comes from and how to get in touch with the right person. With a little investigative work, you will soon find yourself inundated with material and contacts. Who knows? You could find yourself on a float in the next parade!

As crazy as it sounds, ethnic restaurants are also good sources. If an establishment features dancing entertainment, you can usually talk to the performers, and they will be more than happy to tell you where they received their training. Some businesses even offer weekly instruction or audience participation as a promotional gimmick. If you aren't brave enough to put a napkin in your teeth and join in the fun, you can corner the instructor later to inquire about private lessons or independent group sessions. These same entertainers are probably registered with theatrical agencies, and a quick look through the Yellow Pages of the phone book (under the Entertainment classification) will give you the telephone numbers of people who could steer you in the right direction or give you a school referral.

If you are interested in mastering a more obscure dance form, you may have to look under a different heading. Keep that phone book handy and try the listings under Clubs and Associations. You will find that many nationalities have social groups, and within each organization there is bound to be someone who is knowledgeable on dance or who knows a qualified teacher.

Musicians are another good source because, of course, where there is dance, there is music. Good, working ethnic musicians are at a premium, so if you can locate them (through schools, clubs, or agencies) they may be able to put you in touch with the dancers that they accompany. You would be amazed at how well everybody knows each other in "the business."

Many of the traditional educational schools also offer excellent ethnic and folk dance classes. You will find African and folk dance at most colleges and universities, and many offer credit and non-credit courses in a wide variety of dance forms. Some schools even have impressive performing companies, and there are a few major universities that are world renowned for their contributions to ethnic dance.

SQUARE DANCE

Elementary and secondary schools and Park and Recreation departments are great places to look if you are interested in square dance instruction. Classes are available for all ages, and the tuition costs are generally more reasonable than at colleges or private facilities. Square dance is not only mentally challenging, it also provides a good physical workout and promotes strong social skills. Don't you remember how much fun it was to do-si-do around the gym in grade school? If you thought that was great, wait until you try it with a bunch of adults. It's guaranteed to bring a smile to your face!

There are square dance clubs all over the U.S. that not only offer instruction but also provide social activities and workshops on a regular basis. Many of these clubs advertise in square dancing magazines, and you can find copies of these publications at any large library or comprehensive book store.

If you can't locate the relevant names and numbers, try a western apparel store. Though they are few in number, if you can locate one they will be able to give you some leads. Many stores even have public bulletin boards to provide their customers with information on schools, clubs, workshops, and callers. Before you know it, you will be swinging your partner through the hay every Friday night.

INSTRUCTOR QUALIFICATIONS

Now that you have found a class and teacher, how do you know if the instructor is qualified? Again, it would be literally impossible to cover all the dance forms, and each one has its own special requirements. I can, however, offer my opinion as to what you should generally look for in an ethnic or folk dance instructor.

You can't take the history out of the dance, nor can you take the dance out of history. They are tightly interwoven and each is an integral part of the other. It stands to reason that an ethnic or folk class should consist of more than mere movement. The teacher should be knowledgeable not only in the steps but also in their origin and significance to the culture. The ritual and history behind each dance gives it its uniqueness and substance and should be passed on during instruction from teacher to student as a priceless legacy.

Authentic costumes should be introduced, directly if at all possible, or indirectly by the use of pictures, films, or other visual aids. If "props" (i.e., castanets, swords, sticks, hats, etc.) are used, they should be relatively authentic and plentiful. Whenever possible, the teacher should make every attempt to use ethnic music, and it should coincide accurately with each particular dance. Of course there will be times, especially in performance, when more commercial songs are appropriate, but they are still no substitute for authentic accompaniment, and students should be exposed to it sometime during their training.

WARMUP

If the type of dance under consideration requires a lot of physical movement, a warmup should be done at the beginning of class to prevent injury. The teacher should know enough physiology to give a safe pre-dance stretch (see Chapter 9), which can guard against the overdevelopment of leg muscles (a potential danger, particularly in Irish and Scottish dance). I have seen many children end up with huge calf muscles because they were not given proper stretches prior to the abusive, excessive hopping required to master some ethnic styles. Observe your child's class carefully, or if you are the student, let your body be your guide. Class should be fun, and you should not be in constant pain. A little discomfort due to the introduction of unusual movement is to be expected, but continual muscle strain is not. When in doubt, consult a doctor.

SPECIAL CLOTHING

Special clothing during class is another issue. Most instructors don't require any type of specialized dancewear during class; however, the very nature of some dance styles requires clothing that allows freedom of movement or is suggestive of actual ethnic costuming. Spanish dance is one such style that comes to mind. Posture is extremely important in this style, and it is necessary for a teacher to see the body's shape. Form-fitting clothing or traditional dancewear would be appropriate in this case, and I would be very leery of an instructor who allows baggy streetwear in such a class. How can hip movements be monitored in a Tahitian class if they are hidden under loose clothing? How can a teacher of Irish dance see the point of the foot if the student is wearing sneakers? The answer to both of these questions is, of course, they can't.

Remember, a teacher's professional attitude will be picked up by her students as easily as they pick up the steps. A good instructor requires proper clothing and does not allow inappropriate dress because it would be inconsistent with her goals of teaching good, safe dance. If a class doesn't look professional, it probably isn't. Try a different studio or a different dance style. After all, there are many, many to choose from.

WRAP-UP

America is truly a melting pot and a veritable smorgasbord of dance exists within its boundaries. It is all yours for the tasting—from the hot and spicy flamenco to the traditional American square dance. Have fun sampling the cuisine. Bon appetit!

PART IV

Dance for Special People and Groups

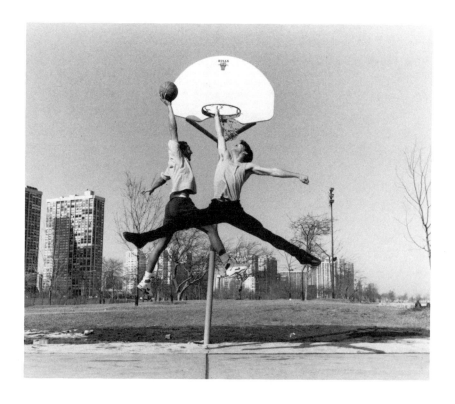

14
Athletes

Those move easiest who have learned to dance.
Alexander Pope

Dancers have finally been recognized as the great athletes they are, and people in the world of sports are realizing the tremendous benefits of including dance as an integral part of their training. Well, it's about time!

It has taken a long time for the mutual admiration society to form, but in many high schools, universities, and professional sport organizations, the dancer and the athlete work together, sharing their expertise. You will find a new respect developing for the body and for the dance. I can truthfully say that any athlete who supplements his or her training with dance will become better at the chosen sport and will gain a whole new appreciation of the mechanics of the human body.

THE VALUES OF DANCE FOR ATHLETES

For the longest time, coaches and trainers stressed only strength, and their means to that end was working relentlessly with weights, aerobic calisthenics, and ballistic bounces (rapid, repetitive movements), especially in the all-male contact sports. Everyone wanted to look like Mr. Universe. What they had overlooked was the need for flexibility and agility—two areas dance embodies. Dancers who have been trained correctly are experts in the art of "warmup." It is this slow, calculated stretch that gives their bodies a defense against injury and affords them lengthy and fruitful careers. Athletes, on the other hand, have relied on external sources to guide them in their percussive "warmups," and the coaches and trainers weren't aware, until recently, that there was a different, safer, and more advantageous approach.

Over the years as dance took its rightful place in academia and was included in the curricula at most major universities, college dance instructors found themselves thrown into the physical education departments. In the long run, it helped the cause. The intimacy of the PE departments forced the dance and athletic instructors to take a serious look at each other. They liked what they saw! Nowadays, if you go into any PE department, you will most likely see dancers working out with weights while the "jocks" are stretching, jumping, and dancing (yes, I said dancing) in the dance classes. It's a marriage made in heaven!

Skater extraordinaire Randy Gardner put it perfectly, "Dance is the basis for every kind of movement ... Dance training early in a career can make you aware of your body and also prevent you from having injuries if you use the proper warm-up techniques."

Dance in Male-Dominated Sports

Though sports such as figure skating and gymnastics were pioneers in incorporating dance into their training, the more "macho" sports are still having a rough time getting it through their thick, muscular skulls. There are famous male sports figures who have come forward, putting up with team ridicule and a lot of snickering, to let the world know the validity of dance for athletes. Former Olympic track star Willie Gault of the L.A. Raiders danced to rave reviews with the Chicago City Ballet when he was one of the Chicago Bears, and Herschel Walker of the Minnesota Vikings took dance and also performed with a regional ballet company. Lynn Swann, formerly of the Pittsburgh Steelers, studied dance for fourteen years and attributed his agility on the field to his dance training. He went one step further (sorry for the pun) and became a trustee of the Pittsburgh Ballet Theatre. And there were more ...

Renowned coach Knute Rockne of Notre Dame believed in the benefits of dance so strongly that he insisted his players take class, and Woody Hayes of Ohio State fame incorporated dance into his training procedures. West Point even had their turn with dance when one-time New York Maritime Academy Welterweight Boxing Champion and now ballet great, Edward Villella, lectured and demonstrated ballet to one hundred of the Army football players. He knew the facts ...

Dance can give athletes agility, endurance, mental alertness, and quickness of movement. It can bring about an increased body awareness and a sense of balance; it can improve jumps and turns and vastly aid flexibility. The risk of injury greatly diminishes when dance stretching techniques are employed, and a good dance warmup helps eliminate muscle and joint soreness.

The problem lies in getting athletes, especially males, to put aside their macho insecurities and get into dance class. The stigma of dance being feminine, or even effeminate, still exists. So how do you get it into the head of an impressionable young boy that dance class can help his diving or track performance or help with his basketball, football, or soccer skills? The only answer is that experience is the best teacher.

The divers at the University of Miami were pretty skeptical until they saw the results. The fundamentals of ballet helped improve the overall "line" of their dives, while the emphasis on proper alignment and centering, combined with turn and jump dissection, polished their techniques. Timing and rhythm improved, and it was all because of ballet. The basketball players at California State University, Long Beach, weren't prepared for the successful encounter that they had either. Modern dance kept them free from groin pulls for an entire season, and their jumps and turns improved by leaps and bounds (I couldn't resist).

My own experience with dance for athletes was when I was student teaching in the dance department at Oakland University in Rochester, Michigan. The baseball coach at the time had observed one of my notorious jazz warmups and, having been plagued with numerous team injuries in the previous season, asked if I would consider giving a stretch class to his players. Quite frankly, I was less than thrilled. The thought of standing in front of a bunch of unwilling jocks in my leotard and trying to get them to cooperate was not my idea of a good time. Much to my surprise, after I got them past the initial shock it proved quite successful. I remember walking into the gym while they all whistled and leered. I knew that the challenge would be getting them to take me seriously. As they chuckled, I forcefully told them, in my drill sergeant voice, to "hit the deck." I further barked that if any of them dared to "mouth off" to me, I'd make them do fifty

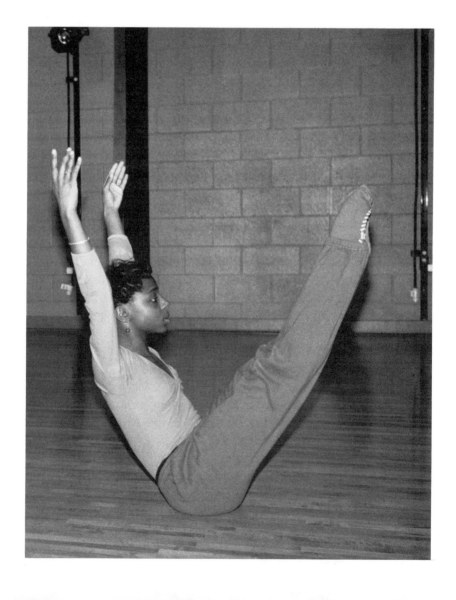

pushups and fifty laps around the gym. A hush settled on the group. Confident with my newfound authority, I proceeded to take them through my most comprehensive stretches. Fearing to look "wimpy," they jumped right in with all the gusto they could muster. (After all, they didn't want to be shown up by a girl.) That's when reality set in. Dance really was tough!

For the next few sessions they silently suffered through the indignity of muscle soreness, but as the days passed, they actually started to enjoy the newfound freedom of muscle and joint flexibility. I will never forget the feeling of accomplishment that I felt when I went to their first game of the season and saw them *voluntarily* sitting in dance second position before the game, doing my stretches and warming up. I am proud to say that there weren't any injuries all season and that I also got a couple of great dinner invitations out of the deal.

Those baseball players would not have taken dance if it had not been required by their coach. Talking your son into lessons may initially require a little of the same arm twisting. After all, society has programmed him into believing that success in sports can be purchased at the local store. The message is that it doesn't take training or body awareness—it only requires the right outfit, equipment, or breakfast food. Commercials featuring big name sports celebrities endorsing everything from sneakers to cereal permeate our lives, taking the responsibility for athletic success off the shoulders of the individual. Is it any wonder that young aspiring athletes, if given the choice, would opt for a pair of $150 autographed sneakers rather than for a semester of supplemental dance classes?

THE EXPERTS' OPINION

Experts are worried about this trend. Michael J. Alter, author of *Sport Stretch* and the *Science of Stretching*, feels that "many athletes (especially young athletes) would better serve themselves if they would spend more time considering and implementing the benefits of a cross-training program such as dance training, rather than wasting both their valuable time and money selecting a certain brand of cross-training shoes that will supposedly make them jump higher or run faster."

As an adult, it's easy to see his point, but as a parent you know, only too well, how unimportant such a rationale is to an adolescent who is consumed with the need to fit in and have the right "look." Guiding an impressionable young lad into supplemental dance classes can be tricky, but one thing that could really help is to find a class with a dynamic male instructor. Though male dance teachers are few and far between, they are out there and it would behoove you to find one. They can be wonderful role models. Time and time again, I have watched the same miracle occur. Once the student discovers the similarity between dance and sports, he rises to the challenge and tackles the complexities of dance with as much enthusiasm as he tackles a wide receiver. It's really an eye opener!

If you can't find a male instructor, don't despair. Many female instructors know how to choreograph generically and are experts in changing the moves to complement their male students. Before signing up, however, scrutinize the teacher's choreography carefully. If the movements look too weak, it would be best to look elsewhere for a more masculine style. It is also helpful if the class is made up entirely of boys (a real rarity) or if there are at least a few other boys in class for camaraderie and friendly competition. Perhaps you could suggest to your son's coach that the whole team could benefit from group dance lessons. As long as you don't get thrown out of his office, it may be a way to provide lots of peer support.

WOMEN ATHLETES

Girls, on the other hand, are a piece of cake. Most are more than willing to take supplementary dance classes. You can, however, make their dance experience even more beneficial by discussing their sports goals with the teacher at the outset. If there are particular results you are looking for, the instructor needs to know that so he or she can develop a game plan. You might even consider private instruction so that the teacher and student can work one on one. Most dance instructors are really open to a challenge. In fact, many, after even a brief exposure to athletes, find themselves in a new career—coaching or choreographing for athletes in competitions.

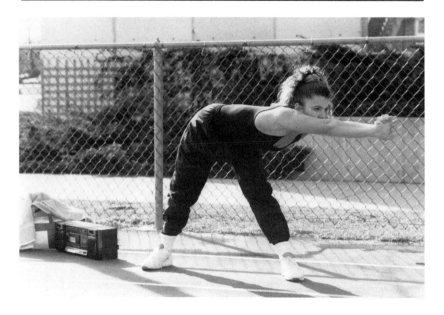

THE PROBLEMS OF DANCE AND SPORTS

Some problems have arisen, however, with this integration of dance and sports. Qualifications and the limits of the dance teacher's participation have become serious issues. A dance teacher supplying choreography for an athlete and working from a purely esthetic standpoint is one thing, but "acting as a coach" is a whole different ball game. Great care must be taken by parents or athletes to be sure that a dance instructor works within the bounds of his or her expertise. Some are indeed highly qualified in not only dance but also in kinesiology and the mechanics of a particular sport; however, most dancers really don't know the intricacies of specific athletic endeavors.

I found this out firsthand when I had my own stint as a choreographer at the National Academy of Skating in Michigan, where I taught ballet, jazz, and stretch to Olympic figure skating hopefuls. Working intimately with the coaches, I learned as much as my students did, and I sure gained a new respect for the coaches and skaters whose dedication got them on the ice at 6:00 a.m. when the rest of the world was having its first cup of coffee. Many a morning was spent freezing my buns off while I ran precariously down the ice and yelled instructions. Those brave kids, my eldest daughter Jamie included, jumped, spun, and fell over and over again for hours until they got it right. (Passion is passion, whether it is in an ice arena or on a Broadway stage.) It quickly became obvious that my knowledge was only a very small part of their intricate training. It took the specialized expertise and gentle hand of the dedicated coaches at the academy to take a skater's passion, mold it, and combine it with my choreography to produce a winner.

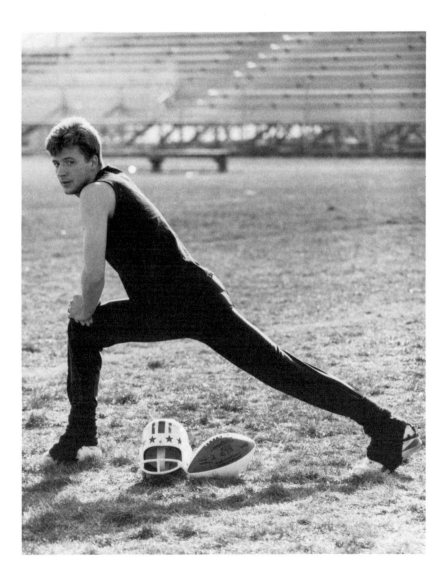

What I'm getting at is that great care should be taken by parents to screen dance instructors to assure that they: (1) know enough information about the specific sport to be beneficial to their child's career; (2) work in conjunction with the acting coach; and (3) don't take over the coaching role unless qualified to do so.

Dr. Martin I. Lorin, Professor of Clinical Pediatrics at Baylor College of Medicine in Houston and author of *Physical Fitness for Children*, stated it quite clearly:

> A coach who is not knowledgeable in the sport may give the youngster improper advice or may fail to recognize danger signals. A coach who is anxious to impress parents, or to chalk up a personal victory, may push a child beyond his or her ability or make a youngster go too far, too early in training. If a youngster is going to participate seriously in a sport, the parents should know something about the coach who will be working with the child. One cannot really judge a coach by his title or degrees alone, nor only by his accomplishments. Rather, one needs to inquire about his personal reputation and his attitudes toward children and toward the sport. A children's coach should certainly have some understanding of the physiology and psychology of the growing child. One needs to watch a coach in action. You are going to be entrusting your child's safety and mental and physical health to this individual. Be sure he or she is a person worthy of that trust.

To put that heavy responsibility on the shoulders of a dance teacher is unrealistic. Dance training is *supplemental* to good, qualified athletic coaching and, if taught by a caring personal instructor can help an athlete have a long, injury-free career and a creative experience, and it can help him realize his dreams.

WRAP-UP

No matter what your athletic goal is, you owe it to yourself or your child to develop it to the best possible potential. Dance can help you get there. Give it a chance and you may find yourself really enjoying it. Who knows? You may even want to trade in your cleats for a pair of dancing shoes.

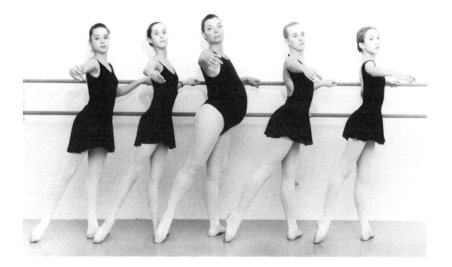

15

Pre- and
Post-Natal Women

Someday the stork may pay a visit
and leave a little souvenir ...
<u>42nd Street</u>

Congratulations! You're going to be a mom! Having had considerable experience in that area (two girls and one boy), I can tell you that not only will your body change but so will your life. It's going to be wonderful! At the time of the writing of this book, my offspring range in age from twenty-two years to five years. Since I danced through all three pregnancies, I feel qualified to put in my two cents worth concerning the benefits of dancing before, during, and after pregnancy. As I am not a doctor, however, I am not qualified to advise you as to the practicality of dance during *your* pregnancy. Instead I'm going to talk about what I do know—the types of dance and the level of exertion each requires. Having this information will help you decide which form of dance is right for you and your child.

MEDICAL CONSIDERATIONS

Each woman is totally different from the next, as is each pregnancy. Every obstetrician/gynecologist whom I talked to basically agreed that the pre- or post-natal activity a woman participates in should depend entirely on the individual mom's and baby's physical condition, as well as on what the mom is used to doing, on a regular basis, in the way of exercise. In a room full of expectant moms, you will find both ends of the spectrum—

those who can do basically anything while they are pregnant and those who should do almost nothing. Most women, however, will fall somewhere in between. I was lucky. I could do anything. I was very young and very healthy with my first child, tap dancing in a Broadway touring show with my second, and still in above-average shape when my son was born two years later. (I wish I could say that now.) *I am not the norm!*

When I look back at my days with the tour of *42nd Street*, I can't believe that I could do that aerobic show ten times a week while being plagued with morning sickness, which in my case was an all-day affair. I would zip onto the stage, tap like a demon possessed, come off, turn green during a lightning fast wig and costume change, grab a gulp of water, smile, and tap back on. INSANITY! My costumes eventually got so tight that the management and I decided it was time for "the chunky one on the end" to go home. I did, but only to start teaching eleven classes a week and taking six. I felt and looked terrific. This pace continued until my "Broadway Baby," Amanda, told me that enough was enough. I stopped dancing for the last two months and was miserable. My body and metabolism were so used to exercise that it was almost like taking away a life support system. I couldn't wait to move again so, two weeks after Amanda Grace was born, I was at the gym.

Being a professional dancer gave me a definite edge. I knew my body so well that I knew its limits. Most people, especially women who are just beginning dance and who are pregnant for the first time, don't know their bodies as well. That is why it is so important to be under a doctor's *constant* supervision and have his or her permission before you even start. The doctor must be made aware of what type of dance you are going to take, what it entails, and how many classes a week you plan to attend. Communication, monitoring, and common sense are the keys.

If you and the baby have been given a clean bill of health, *moderate* dance instruction and stretch can be just the ticket. It can help you look and feel great; keep you mentally and socially stimulated; make things easier before, during, and after birth; and it's also a lot more fun than plain, boring exercise. So go ahead and buy yourself a really, really, big T-shirt; have the words "I'm not fat, I'm pregnant!" imprinted on the front, and indulge yourself. You will not have much time to do it later.

THE RIGHT TEACHER

The most important element in a successful pre- or post-natal dance class is the teacher. The instructor must, first, know that you are pregnant (you would be amazed at how many students don't tell their teachers until it becomes really obvious) and second, be knowledgeable enough in physiology and kinesiology to know what stretches or moves could be dangerous — or should care enough to be willing to find out. Since it is not reasonable to expect dance teachers to be expert obstetricians, you will have to take the initiative and ask your doctor about specific hazardous positions or activities (lying on your back, long periods of aerobic movement, etc.) and any warning signals that you should watch out for (dizziness, bleeding, etc.). Always be your own monitor. Learn to take your pulse and get your doctor's recommendation as to the limits to which you should push yourself. Usually it will only take a little basic knowledge to be able to adapt to a regular dance class. Before you know it, you will be "just another dancer" discovering the beauty of your own movement.

I used to love to watch the transformation. Every time I saw a pregnant lady in one of my classes, it would warm the cockles of my heart. Nothing is as cute as a waddling mama-to-be in a bulging leotard wearing tap shoes or a tutu. Of course, I am one of those people who firmly believe women look more beautiful when they are pregnant. I love watching them grow and glow, enjoying their bodies as they forget, at least for an hour or so, that they have been invaded by an internal place-kicker who gives them heartburn and makes life uncomfortable and sound sleep impossible. They are a joy to behold! Whether they were experienced dancers who were still dancing rings around most of their peers or raw beginners who were looking for an alternative to bland pre- and post-natal exercise classes, one fact remained the same—they were having a great time and were doing something beneficial and of lasting value for themselves and their babies.

WHAT'S RIGHT FOR YOU?

Now that you have decided to join the ranks and become a dancing duo, what type of dance would you like to take? Most forms can be attempted at a *beginning* level while pregnant; however, types that involve a lot of hopping or jumping (some ethnic styles) should be avoided until after the baby is born. Again, it all depends on what condition you are in and the teacher and her particular style and method of teaching. For instance, some tap teachers' styles are smooth and fluid, while others have you hip-hopping all over the place. You will need to observe the class that you are considering to determine whether it looks like something you could safely handle. Doctors today are a lot more liberal than they used to be when it comes to bouncing and aerobic activity, but there is still a limit to the amount of jarring a baby can take. If you feel that modifying your moves to accommodate your condition would not let you benefit sufficiently from the class, maybe you need to make another choice.

BEGINNER BALLET AND MODERN

Probably the two easiest dance styles, in terms of least aerobic movement, are beginner ballet and modern dance. Most of the moves are slow and controlled and give you time to adjust your body and alignment. There are also some real additional benefits to these classes. The emphasis on posture and alignment can help alleviate backaches, and circulation may be improved, which could help ward off those nasty leg cramps. You will also feel a little more feminine and graceful (at least at the outset). There will be a few minor obstacles to overcome—getting your leg up on the barre will be tricky, and your newly developed breasts will get in the way of certain arm movements, but hey, everybody needs a little challenge. Anyway, it will be well worth it.

JAZZ

Jazz is another fun class to try. It affords many of the same benefits as ballet and modern with the addition of an aerobic workout. The pre-dance stretch will probably be more strenuous, so the whole body will get toned. Be sure to keep monitoring your blood pressure as the "combinations" will move faster and require more effort, but if the teacher is qualified, there should not

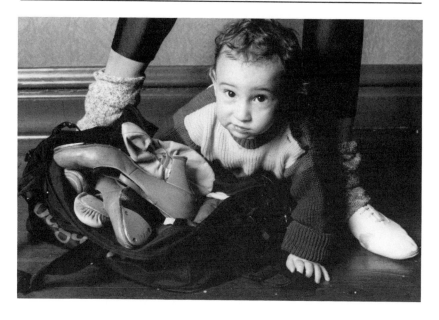

be any added risks in taking this type of class. In fact, jazz classes have the added benefit of stress relief. The feeling of freedom that comes with the movements and the use of contemporary music will make you "get down" and relax in no time.

CLASSES TO AVOID

What about social dance? Well, unfortunately you might find that you will want to hold off on lessons of this type for nine months or so. Ballroom dance, though a great way to get out with your husband, is really not a practical choice once your belly starts expanding. It's hard to work as a close couple when "something has come between you." After the baby is born, however, it's a perfect way to get exercise, have a weekly date with your neglected spouse, and put some romance back into your life. Get a sitter, grab your heels, and go lambada for awhile. It's guaranteed to be a welcome relief from dirty diapers and spit up!

The ethnic dance styles are probably also better put "on the back burner" while you have a bun in the rest of the oven. You may be able to find a kilt with an elastic waist, a maternity flamenco dress, or an expandable hula skirt, but I do think that belly dancing is out of the question. Of course, that's only my opinion. Maybe having a big belly makes you better at it. Who knows?

WRAP-UP

Check with your doctor, use your head as well as your body, grab your dance bag, and go. In nine months, you will be carrying a diaper bag and a new baby instead. Perhaps your child will someday be a Broadway star. Maybe osmosis really works!

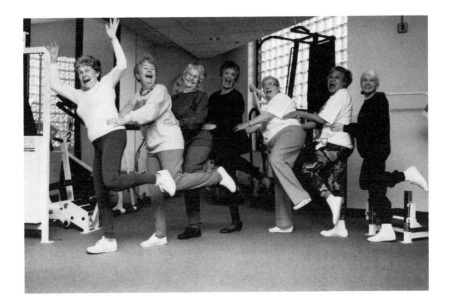

16
Senior Citizens

Gotta move 'cause time is a wastin'
There's sure a lot of livin' to do!
<u>Bye</u>, <u>Bye</u> <u>Birdie</u>

Whoever coined the phrase, "You are only as old as you feel," really hit the nail on the head. Old age may be only a state of mind, but that state of mind is, in reality, directly connected to the condition of the body. In order to keep feeling physically young, you have to keep physically fit and exercise. There is not a more enjoyable way to accomplish both than by dancing. Not only will you feel stronger and remain flexible, but your mind will get a workout as well. On top of it all, your heart will stay in shape, your balance will improve, depression and stress will vanish, and you will meet a whole lot of new friends. How can you possibly resist?

Senior classes are offered through recreation and community centers, at dance studios, through continuing education at schools and universities, through church groups, and at many residential facilities for the elderly. You can learn to mambo, tap, pirouette, square dance, or "boogie." The possibilities are endless. It is all there for the picking. You just have to want to dance and have enough guts to GO FOR IT!

One of the most difficult things for seniors to do is to take advantage of all the recreational opportunities available. It is really hard to take that first step and get involved. I promise you, however, that once you do, you will see that the "golden years" are indeed filled with fun and excitement. You have one of the most valued commodities in our society—time. I envy you. I wish that I could find the time with my busy schedule to go to dance class a couple of times a week. It would be pure heaven. Once you take the initiative and discover the benefits of dance, I promise that you will be on cloud nine too!

CHECK OUT AVAILABLE CLASSES

Go to your local community center or YMCA and see what classes are available. In fact, grab your spouse, friend, or neighbor and make them go with you. Think of it as an adventure. Signing up for class with a pal can really make that first move a lot less painful. It is so much more fun to go with a "buddy" because it helps break the ice during those awkward first sessions and can motivate you to get to class on a regular basis. Consistency is the key to a successful dance experience. If you are to get anything out of a seniors' dance class, you have to attend at least two or three times a week, and you must be committed to your exercise goal. On those days when you just don't feel like going or you have the blues, a buddy can work miracles in getting you to class. I will let you in on a little secret—even the professionals have a hard time getting their rumps to class. Once there, however, you will soon forget why you procrastinated, and you will get drawn into the movement. You will have a ball. It will probably even become an exciting biweekly social event. Before you grab onto the conga line, however, let's talk about precautions, special teacher qualifications, and the elements that should be present in a safe dance facility.

YOUR PHYSICAL CONDITION

Even if you are in tiptop physical condition, you *must* consult a doctor *before* you jump into any program. Even if the instructor is knowledgeable in the specifics of dance instruction for the over fifty-five crowd, there can be dangers if you don't know yourself and your own limitations, and if you don't inform the teacher of any legitimate medical concerns.

After your doctor's go-ahead and *before* the first class, it is mandatory that you discuss any serious health problems or relevant medications with your instructor. For instance, if you are taking a specific medication to slow down your heart rate, you won't want to be in a class that moves so fast it will speed it up.

If you have diabetes, the sense of feeling in your feet could be impaired, which could lead to balance or coordination problems. A teacher needs to be made aware of this possibility. Arthritis sufferers should be very cautious about the types of stretches that they do. There should be no bouncing or sharp moves, which could seriously injure susceptible joints. Have an open and frank discussion with the teacher beforehand and don't be shy about asking about her qualifications and background. Has she ever taught seniors before? Is she enthusiastic, and does she look fun? And don't forget the most important question of all—is she CPR-certified (in case the fun gets out of hand). After signing up, don't forget to give them any and all emergency phone numbers (relatives, doctors, hospital). An experienced teacher of seniors should ask for this information before the session begins, but if she forgets, take the initiative and furnish a complete list.

CLASS STRUCTURE

It is also really important to ask how the class will be structured and paced. First, will there be enough breaks? In talking to experts who teach senior classes, they all agree that the biggest problem is overenthusiasm on the part of the students. They don't know when to stop! Most are so full of spunk and get-up-and-go that they forget the body may not want to keep up the pace. As noted Chicago dance therapist Gina Demos so eloquently put it, "Students have to be given 'permission to be cautious.'" In other words, they have to know that it is OK to go slow and take breaks. The instructor should encourage spontaneous breaks, and monitoring by the individual should be stressed. In fact, rest periods should be scheduled into the dance session at various intervals, and students should be taught how to take their own pulse. A good teacher will even incorporate it into the class. Staying on top of things and learning to pace yourself could prevent a potentially dangerous situation from arising, but don't put the entire burden on the teacher. She can only do so much. When it comes right down to it, you are the only one who can tell when you have had enough, if it hurts, or if you need a break. When you are feeling the warning signals—stop! Be your own internal monitor and don't push it!

PACE OF THE CLASS

The pace of the class is the next important element. Ask about the class content. Great care should be taken by the instructor to ensure that there is an adequate *slow* warmup at the beginning of class, followed by a more vigorous dance "peak" (which is progressive in its intensity), and a slow "cool down" stretching session at the end. Be sure that the class is not too strenuous. If everything sounds great, then the next step is to check out the facility itself.

THE FACILITY

Most seniors' classes are offered in less than perfect dance conditions since many take place in community centers or in large "meeting rooms." Because of this, it is crucial that you find a facility with a safe floor (see Chapter 3). Carpeting is common, and it is acceptable *if* it works with the type of dance you are studying. Let's face it, you can't tap dance on carpet!

The room should be clean, pleasant, and free of structural obstructions (pillars, poles, etc.), and it should be adequate for the size of the class. It should have good lighting and ventilation. Fans and/or air conditioning are mandatory in the summer since seniors are more susceptible to heat stroke. For the same reason, the heat should be consistent in the winter months and not so oppressive as to elevate body temperatures dangerously. Rest rooms and changing areas should be *adjacent* to the dance room, and there should be enough seating so that all students can take a breather.

The class itself should be moderate in size so that the instructor can monitor each student individually. This is important. If you feel that you will be getting lost in the crowd because there are too many students in the class, then you probably will. Suggest splitting the class in two or starting a second class or look for another class. Get your money's worth. You deserve it.

DANCEWEAR

Everything looks perfect and you can't wait to start! What do you wear? Clothing *is* an important issue. Most seniors don't feel comfortable in traditional dancewear so, unless your instructor insists on it, loose activewear (sweat pants and shirts, shorts, T-shirts, etc.) is more than appropriate. Be sure that it is lightweight and not restrictive, so you can swing those hips freely. If you are going to change at the facility, you might want to invest in an inexpensive dance bag. This way you can keep all your things together, including your valuables, and take them into class with you. It's a lot easier dealing with one bag than trying to juggle a purse, clothing, accessories, and shoes all at the same time.

FOOTWEAR AND OTHER NECESSITIES

Footwear is another serious consideration. Your choice of shoes should be made on an individual basis. The amount of support you will require depends entirely on your own body and needs. Don't skimp! Be sure that whatever you choose is appropriate for the class and has a sole that is safe for the flooring in the facility. Your doctor or teacher should be able to advise you accordingly.

No tight or elastic stockings or garters should be worn. They could severely inhibit blood flow. Just keep it "au naturel."

Here are a few more things that you will want to take to class. Have enough liquid handy (one of those plastic athletic squeeze bottles works great) to keep replenishing your system because older adults need additional liquid, and exercise will increase your body's demand. Keeping some healthy snacks on hand is also a good idea. In fact, have each student take a turn bringing a favorite snack to pass around. You might even come away with a few good recipes!

WRAP-UP

If you choose wisely and use common sense, you will come away with a lot more than that. You will feel great, look great, and have a great time. You will feel confident with your choice so that you can relax and enjoy it to its fullest. Kick those heels up and have fun! Let your inhibitions melt away and let your fantasies come true. What are you waiting for? It's never too late to let the good times roll!

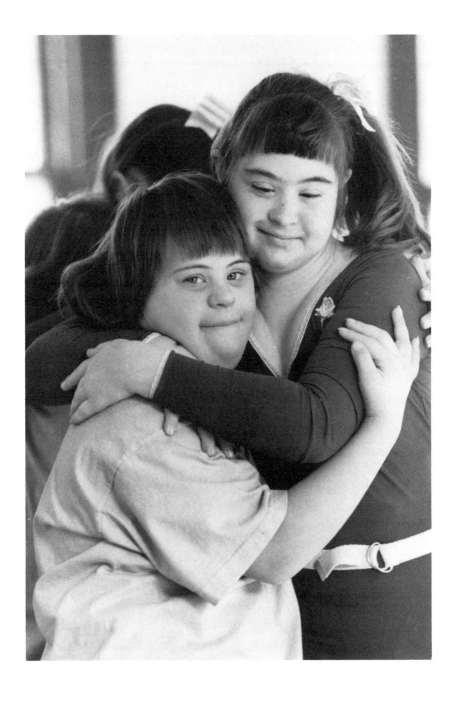

17
Dancers with Disabilities

But oh, she dances such a way!
No sun upon an Easter day
Is half so fine a sight!
Sir John Suckling

When I began researching classes for "special people," it became quite evident that there is a real deficit of classes in this area. The field of dance therapy is in its infancy, and most teachers who do not possess this specialized training are refusing to accept students who have disabilities. The reasons are unclear. It could be that studio owners fear the added financial liability as insurance rates climb, lawsuits abound, and insurance carriers advise them against taking risks. Perhaps they feel that classes of this type would be difficult and unprofitable, or maybe they just don't want to get involved. Whatever the case, people with even minimal disabilities are finding it difficult, if not impossible, to find dance instruction outside of the appropriate institutional facilities.

There are, however, instructors who are pioneers in trying to mainstream deaf, blind, or Down syndrome students into their regular classes, or who have seen the growing need and demand for isolated classes for these individuals in a studio setting, and who are boldly filling these needs. I believe that the physically and mentally impaired have the right to the same dance opportunities as you and I. Dance helps them physically, emotionally, and socially. It can increase body awareness, help with coordination and muscle strength, improve social skills, boost self-esteem, and bring about a major feeling of accomplishment. It can work miracles. Dance can, however, if taught by an uneducated, insensitive instructor, or if taught in the wrong setting (mainstreaming vs. special classes), become a nightmare and a setback rather than positive stimulation. You have to make your placement decision carefully if you want the experience to be successful, and it may take quite a long time to find a class. You might even have to organize one yourself. Whatever you decide, just be sure to study all the facts before you make a choice. In today's dance world, you basically have only three options: (1) mainstreaming your child into a regular dance class at a dance facility; (2) finding or organizing a special class in a regular dance facility, which will be made up of only disabled students; or (3) enlisting the services of a private dance therapist.

MAINSTREAMING

Let's discuss mainstreaming first. I talked to many teachers and therapists who are actively working in the field, and almost all agree that the success rate of mainstreaming, especially for the severely disabled, is minimal at best. Here is what they told me . . .

Everything hinges on the individual child—his or her specific problems, personality, and unique physical, behavioral, and mental limitations. Mainstreaming your child into a regular class at a dance facility affects not only the child but the rest of the students as well. Sometimes it can be an eye-opening, positive experience for all concerned but, unfair as it may be, most of the time it just does not work. The students and their "paying parents" resent the interruptions and the inconvenience of having a child in class whose level (mental and/or physical) is not equal to the rest of the members of the group. In the case of a deaf dancer who may require the assistance of an interpreter, the students, especially younger ones, find the interpreter distracting. The deaf student's attention has to bounce back and forth from the signer to the teacher to the mirror, and the tendency is for the movement to win out, thus making the instructional experience incomplete and less than successful. If the child is blind, the other students become inhibited with their own movements because they fear getting too close to the sightless student and possibly getting in his way or frightening him. In addition, the "normal" vocalizing or inconsistent behavioral problems of some impaired people can be unsettling to the other students who don't understand them or their impairment. If the class is made up of very young children, it can actually frighten them and make them drop out of class. In severe impairment cases, I think that everyone would be happier if there were a specific class where all the disabled with the same impairment could dance together.

A SPECIAL CLASS

This is your second option—a special class. I feel that this type of instruction should be available for all people with impairments in every community. Unfortunately, studio owners just don't want to offer these types of classes. As daunting as it might be, you are going to have to take the bull by the horns and talk them into it. It is not going to be easy.

First, you will have to locate a reputable studio, then a willing, appropriate teacher at the facility and—here's the difficult part—you will have to have enough students to offer them so that they will profit from the class. Perhaps through support groups or other activities you have met parents whose children would benefit from group dance instruction. If so, use this to your advantage. Studio owners have their own reality to deal with. There are only so many class times available (especially after school), and each time period is potential income. If you can hand the owner a new class, it could definitely sway him to try something innovative. If the owner agrees to your proposal, then the next step is finding out which of his staff is best suited and willing to teach this type of class.

INSTRUCTOR QUALIFICATIONS

What specific requirements should a dance instructor for the handicapped possess? The first thing to look for is a willingness to get involved. If the owner has to force someone to teach the class, you don't want that person! The teacher you are looking for must be sensitive, patient, and enthusiastic, and must want to communicate not only with the students but with parents. The teacher must also be realistic in the goals for each student, enjoy teaching beginners, and be willing to get to know each student and the scope of his or her impairment intimately. Perhaps the teacher could enlist the aid of regular students who could volunteer to work on a one-to-one "buddy system." This assistance would provide peer contact and positive role models for the disabled, while giving the regular students a whole new insight into the impaired, themselves, and movement. Structuring the class in this manner would also help to take away the stigma of being "different" and would let the handicapped person have a sense of belonging to the rest of the facility.

COMMUNICATION

Communication is the next consideration. If the students are deaf and if sign language is needed, the instructor must be willing to learn to sign visually and/or be able to relate through tactile signing. The teacher must also know the scope of each person's deafness, so that he may manipulate sound in the class to benefit each individual. Having the knowledge to be able to position people correctly to help them pick up vibrations or beats is mandatory, and knowing acceptable decibel levels can keep a pupil free from additional auditory injury.

DISCIPLINE

And what about discipline? The instructor must know what he or she is getting into and should talk openly with the parents about their child and the proper way to react if he becomes withdrawn, uncooperative, overexcited, or loses his attentiveness.

PRIVATE CLASSES

As you well know, there is a lot involved in teaching the disabled, and the teacher must be made aware of the extra effort it will require. Once established, however, a dance class for the disabled can provide immense benefits for the students, their peers, and the teacher, and if nurtured will grow and prosper for many years to come. The hard part is getting it started. If I had my way, all studios would offer special classes for the impaired. Unfortunately, in the immediate future it just is not going to happen. With some perseverance on your part, however, these types of classes could become available to all who need them in your area.

Your third option is to have a licensed dance therapist teach your child either in a private studio setting (of which there are only a handful) or in a residential institutional facility. Almost all facilities for the disabled offer some type of physical therapy. It can be administered by a regular physical therapist, a music therapist, or a dance therapist. If dance is not being offered in your facility, you will have to take the initiative.and go to the administrator and suggest it. Chances are that if the facility has a music therapist, she is already incorporating some dance or movement into their programs or would be more than happy to give it a try. Putting a dance therapist on staff, however, is a whole different ball game. Suggest that a therapist be brought in on a trial basis or as a guest teacher. Once the administrator sees the results, the benefits of this type of therapy will become more evident. Who knows? You may start a whole new program.

As far as private dance therapists are concerned, they are very few in number. Most work through clinics, psychiatric hospitals, correctional facilities, developmental centers, or special schools, but there are a few who operate private dance facilities for therapeutic movement or who rent space in regular dance studios to work with clients. These innovators offer a valuable service to the emotionally and physically disabled, and if you can find one you will be glad you did. Be sure, however, that the therapist is registered with the American Dance Therapy Association (D.T.R.), which will mean that she is qualified in dance therapy, has a dance background, and has a master's degree. Always do your homework to make sure that the instructor did hers!

WRAP-UP

Whatever path you decide to take, be realistic in your expectations. There will be many setbacks along the way, but the rewards of dance for the disabled are too great to be measured and should not be ignored. Remember, anyone can dance and should have the opportunity to learn. Each person's dance is his own.

PART V

Words of Wisdom

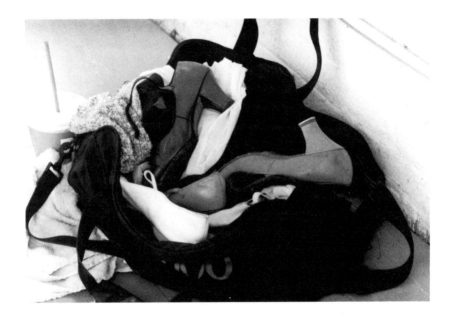

18
Advice to the Serious Student

Those who dance are thought mad by those who hear not the music.
Unknown

The minute I put on my first pair of tap shoes at the Dickerman Dance Studio in Farmington, Michigan, I knew I had to be a dancer. I had no choice. There was nothing else in the world that I wanted to do. At that moment, within the confines of those four cinder block walls, the realization of why I was put on this earth hit me square between the eyes. I was going to be a dancer!

Everyone around me thought I was nuts! How could a five year old know her destiny? Stranger still, why would she ever pick such an odd career? I didn't pick it. It picked me. All the ridicule in the world was not about to change my mind. That's when I met my mentor and first teacher, a red-headed fireball named Virginia Dickerman. Mrs. D's passion and expertise nurtured my love for tap as she incessantly drilled me on every nuance of my craft. I owe her a great deal. Thanks to Mrs. D., I had the necessary tap skills to land two national tours of *42nd Street* and realize my dreams. Every time I tapped my rump off in my platinum wig on those infamous oversized dimes to the strains of "We're in the Money," I thought of her. Thanks, Mrs. D. It wasn't easy but it was a hell of a ride!

If you too are driven to pursue dance as a career, you have chosen to maneuver down a very bumpy, winding road. Don't get me wrong, it will be well worth the trip, but you will have to deal with the detours and roadblocks. Here is the bottom line: *You must want to dance more than anything else in the world and must be prepared to be completely devoted to your craft and goals in order to gain the skills you will need to "make it" in the professional world.* You must be DEDICATED! Without dedication, you haven't got a chance. It really is a jungle out there.

THE RIGORS OF DANCE TRAINING

As a student in training, you will have to go to class religiously and as your ability increases, that usually means *daily* class. Stretching and dancing will become as normal and necessary to your body as eating or sleeping, and the studio will become your home. Your dance bag will become your closet and your refrigerator and, in many instances, your pillow. Your life will consist of school and dance class, dance class and school. You will not have time for many extracurricular activities. Your social calendar will be filled with workshops, studio performances, and washing your tights and leotards out in the sink every night. (Pretty glamorous, huh?) Most of the time, you will be too exhausted to do even that.

As you become an adult and your training accelerates, the demands of the real world will make matters more complex. You will have to support yourself while you train and try to hold down a job (probably waiting tables) while you continue to immerse yourself in classes. In your spare time (in your dreams), you will have to squeeze in as many voice and acting lessons as humanly possible to increase your marketability. If you want a musical theater career, you will have to work to become a "triple threat"—one who can dance, sing, *and* act. You'll find it is necessary to become competent in all these areas to give yourself a wider range of employment opportunities. (If you don't possess these skills, you will find yourself spending more time in the unemployment line than in the chorus line.) On top of all this, you will have to take part in as many unpaid performances as you can (to get experience), attend as much theater as you can afford (to become knowledgeable of the market), and find time for your family and social life. GOOD LUCK!

APPLYING YOUR SKILLS

Once you have honed your skills and figured out how to manage it all, it gets worse. Now you have to learn how to *apply* your skills and make some money with them. You will have to know where to find out about auditions, what acceptable industry-quality headshots (photos) are and where to get them taken and duplicated, how to put together a typeset résumé, how to pick appropriate vocal selections and sheet music for each audition and find and memorize monologues, learn what to wear to auditions, and become knowledgeable about theatrical unions. Sound a little overwhelming? Well, it is!

But wait—now comes the really, REALLY hard part ... the rejections! Audition after audition, rejection after rejection, no callbacks, much less a contract. How will you keep going when no one will give you a job? PERSEVERANCE, my friend, with a capital P. You just keep trying. Remember way back at the beginning when you searched your soul and said that you didn't want to do anything else with your life but dance? Well, if you keep the faith—you will. If you want it badly enough and if you have the skills, you will make it. Believe in yourself when no one else does and keep plugging. Believe me, it will be ambrosia when you taste the fruits of your labors.

I am going to leave you with words of advice and wisdom from some highly respected and successful people in the business. Listen to them well. They've been there.

GOOD LUCK ON YOUR JOURNEY! I HOPE THAT YOU DANCE YOUR LIFE AWAY!

WORDS FROM THE PROS

"It takes 100% dedication and love for the art. There is no more difficult a career. So, if you don't love it more than anything, you may find the obstacles too hard to endure."

Juliet Prowse

"Study with the best. Do some asking and talking and find out. Audit the classes and find the teacher and technique for *you*."

Paul Geraci—*Gypsy, Anything Goes, Give My Regards to Broadway, A Chorus Line*; films: *Vice Versa, Ferris Bueller's Day Off*

"Keep an open mind. Read and view everything you can get your hands on that relates to the area that you are headed for."

Becky Garrett—*Blackstone, Annie*; film: *Splash*

"If you want to dance seriously, *do*. You must think about it day and night, dream about it—desire it. If you are not serious, if you have any doubt, reconsider your priorities."

Christa Justus—*Les Miserables*

"Take class as much as possible — for building strength and stamina. Ask your teacher if you can demonstrate and/or assist lower level classes. Never underestimate going back to basics."

Rebecca Timms—*Cats, West Side Story, Guys & Dolls*; film: *Flashdance*

"Be patient. Be precise. *Listen* and think about corrections. Spend time on your own working on what you've learned and are learning about your own body and its own unique way of moving. Love what you're doing. If you don't—don't bother."

Doug Okerson—*42nd Street, Evita*; film: *Annie*; TV: "Loveboat," "General Hospital"; Club acts: Perry Como, Debbie Reynolds, Suzanne Somers, The Osmonds

"Do not dance *only*. If you have given serious consideration to pursuing a career in performance, take acting, take singing. Give yourself some options. The more you have to offer, the more you will be rewarded by doing what you do for a living. Set goals for yourself and go after them. WANT IT."

Neal Hopkins—Singer/Dancer: Bally's Grand (Reno, NV), Royal Caribbean Lines, Norwegian Caribbean Lines; films: *The Wizard, Kill Me Again*

"Stay in shape. Eat well. Don't do drugs. Your body is your instrument and *must* be in top form."

Deanna Dys—*Legs Diamond, Meet Me in St. Louis, My One and Only, 42nd Street*

"Avoid studios that have lots of recitals. They tend to just teach the choreography for the show and don't spend enough time teaching technique and performance skills. Follow your instincts. When something feels terribly wrong, it probably is."

Trudi Green—*42nd Street, Sarava, Seesaw, Promises, Promises,*

Hellzapoppin, Hello, Dolly; films: *All That Jazz, Music Box, Godfather II*

"Look for a studio that has a proven track record for developing working professionals."

Chris Peterson—*On Your Toes, Anything Goes, 42nd Street, Sugar Babies;* films: *Field of Dreams, Working Girl, Fatal Attraction, January Man;* TV: "One Life to Live," "Law and Order"

"Study from as many teachers as possible to get a feeling for many different styles of dance. Teachers with professional experience I feel are the best ... a teacher who loves teaching and has patience."

Michelle O'Steen—*Gypsy, Sweet Charity, Anything Goes, 42nd Street, On Your Toes*

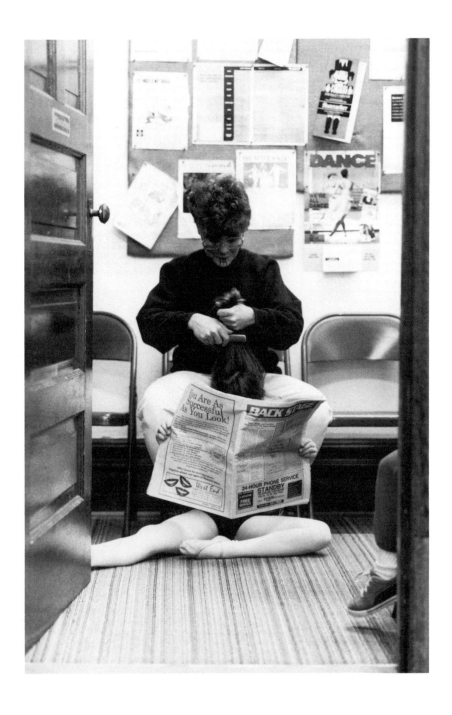

19
Student and Parent Responsibilities

I have just given you a whole book on how to find the right dance class and teacher for you or your child, but you won't succeed in even the most perfect situation or with the most gifted teacher if you don't do *your* part. Pardon one last pun, but ... it takes two to tango! You as a student have certain responsibilities. If the student is not an adult, then those responsibilities fall on the shoulders of the parents. It's all really rather simple. Get your money's worth by observing what I like to call the *4 P's of Responsibility:* Promptness, Preparedness, Practice, and Patience.

PROMPTNESS

Promptness is easy. Be on time for class. Every moment, stretch, and movement are important, and you owe it to yourself and your classmates to be punctual and attend every class. Nothing is more aggravating than having to waste class time repeating information because someone walks in late or because a student's attendance is sporadic. If you aren't there, you will miss something that could come back to haunt you later on, so *get to class and get there on time.*

PREPAREDNESS

When you get to class you have to be prepared. Keep all your dance attire and shoes in a dance bag, and be sure to bring all the essentials with you to class. A special bag also helps keep your things together at the dance facility and avoids confusion. When there are twenty ballerinas in one class, and they are all wearing the same thing, and there are twenty pairs of pink ballet shoes floating around, it sure helps to have yours labeled and in your bag. Allow enough time to get dressed *before* class or have your dancewear on underneath your street clothes. If class is to start at 3:00 p.m. then you should be dressed, hair pinned up, and shoes on, *ready to dance* at 3:00, not waltzing through the door at 2:59. Why waste even five minutes of your class? Every minute is precious.

PRACTICE

Being prepared also means being ready mentally. That brings me to the third P—practice. You are always going to run into those annoying people who have the uncanny ability to pick up steps immediately and who can retain them without effort. Those kinds of "goody two shoes" make the rest of us feel totally stupid and inadequate. In actuality, however, most people need some (if not a lot of) practice between classes to strengthen their skills and to cement things into their memory. The amount of practice you will require depends on many different factors— your individual ability, the degree of difficulty of the material, the time pressures of performance, and the capacity of your memory skills. There should, however, be some attempt at review or some drilling if the student expects to progress and not pull down the level for the rest of the class.

You can make this process a lot less painful if you have the right supplies and your own little space to help you. How can you practice tap sounds on carpet? How can you see your arm movements without a mirror? It's really quite simple to take care of these problems. A sheet of plywood that can be stored under your bed becomes a great dance surface when pulled out. An inexpensive full-length mirror (which can be stored on top of the plywood) can be propped up nearby to check body movements. The back of any sturdy straight back or folding chair makes a great ballet barre. Add some practice music, which you can buy or tape from class, and you're all set. There is no reason to procrastinate!

It is also helpful, if not essential, to write down the steps that you learn, and this should be done as soon as possible after class. You would be amazed at how quickly your brain will forget and how reassuring it will be to know that you have notes to help you between classes. Write the material down in your own words so that you can decipher it. Don't worry about specific terms unless you are sure you know what they mean. After all, these notes are for you, not for anyone else. If your child is the student, ask her to show you what she learned. Even though you may not be taking dance, you will be able to help her write things down to remember the sequence. This testing will also let you monitor her progress and determine whether she needs additional help.

PATIENCE

The last P, patience, is the hardest. Give yourself and the teacher time. It is going to be a slow process, and there may be many times when you will get frustrated and want to give up. Hang in there and before you know it, everything will start falling into place. Try a specific dance style for a minimum of six months to a year before you throw in the towel. It will take at least that long for you or your child to get a true sense of the movement and the teacher's style.

While I am on the subject of patience, a few words of caution are in order. Parents, don't burn your child out with too many stimuli! Attempting a variety of different dance forms at the same time can be really confusing to a very young child, and you will see more enthusiasm and success if you initially enroll your child in one type of dance. Many teachers out there are going to hate me for this advice, but I believe that more children would continue in dance if they were not pushed into it so fast in the beginning and if they didn't take combination classes (half tap, half ballet). All along I have been preaching quality— not quantity. As a child progresses out of the beginning level classes, it becomes easier to incorporate different types of dance into the repertoire. She has plenty of time to master all the different forms, and achieving a modicum of success in one of the more basic styles (i.e., ballet or modern) actually aids in the "digestion" of another kind of dance. Slow down for your child's sake!

KNOWING WHERE TO DRAW THE LINE

While I am talking to you parents, I have to talk to you about the time when your responsibility stops. Let's assume that you have taken my advice and found a great teacher for your child, you are comfortable with his or her competence, and you are willing to follow the 4 P's of Responsibility. How much more involvement should you have in your child's dance training? The answer is, almost none! My answer may sound harsh, but I have always believed that if you want something done right, hire an expert and then leave him or her alone to do the job.

There is nothing more irritating to a dance instructor than a parent who keeps sticking her nose into class, demanding things, and basically making everybody's life miserable. The teacher can't do her job effectively, the child is embarrassed and resentful, and the morale of the entire class can be compromised. DON'T BE A STAGE MOTHER OR FATHER! Trust your teacher to do what is right. After all, you read an entire book on the subject to educate yourself before you made your choice, and you have made a good one. Of course, you should always watch out of the corner of your eye for anything that looks suspicious, but I'll bet that you won't see a thing. You have done your homework, gotten an A-plus on the course, and the teacher and facility have made the grade. The only job left for you is to be encouraging and positive—applauding every little triumph. It's time to bask in the light of your child's success and marvel at the joy of dance.

References

Averyt, Anne C. *Successful Aging*. New York: Ballantine Books, 1987.

Chicago Tribune, September 29, 1986 (Sec. 5): 1,3.

Freeman, Roger D. *Can't Your Child Hear?* Baltimore: University Park Press, 1977.

Greenhill, Janet. "Annette Lewis—The Dancing Jocks of Habersham County." *Dance Teacher Now* (September 1990): 15-20.

Griffith, Betty R. "Modern Dance for Basketball Players." *JOPERD* (May 1981): 32-34.

Lance, James. "Practicing for Touchdowns." *JOPERD* (May 1981): 38.

Leventhal, Marcia B. "Dance Therapy." NDA Fact Sheet, National Dance Association.

Nevell, Richard. *A Time To Dance — American Country Dancing From Hornpipes To Hot Hash*. New York: St. Martin's Press, 1977.

The New York Times, February 8, 1980 (Sec. 1): 23.

The New York Times, September 7, 1981 (Sec. 3): 14.

Pruett, Diane Milhan. "Ballet for Divers." *JOPERD* (May 1981): 34-37.

——. "Male High School Athletes in Dance Classes." *JOPERD* (May 1981): 43-45.

Rappoport, Ken. *Wake Up The Echoes*. Huntsville, AL: Strode Publishing Inc., 1975.

Scott, Eileen P., James E. Jan, and Roger D. Freeman. *Can't Your Child See?* Baltimore: University Park Press, 1977.

About the Author

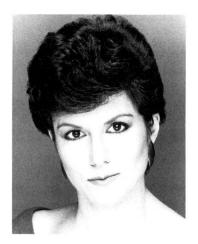

Barbara Early has devoted over thirty-five years to dance and has danced, performed, and choreographed in almost every medium of entertainment from stage to screen. She has danced in Broadway National tours, regional theater, dinner theater, and summer stock; revues, industrial shows, and films; fashion shows and TV commercials, but she feels that her biggest accomplishments are her long list of successful students. Having been a dedicated dance educator and owner of three professional dance schools, as well as a guest teacher or artist-in-residence at numerous colleges, schools, and studios, she has given hundreds of students the tools to go on to careers on Broadway, in dance companies, in film, and on TV. Barbara knows firsthand what makes a superb teacher, a safe studio, and a great class, and what dance can do for students of all ages, levels, and aspirations. She hopes that her knowledge will help you have a wonderful, safe, enlightening dance experience!

Index